Prevention

STRETCH

AWAY PAIN

Prevention

STRETCH

AWAY PAIN

5 Minutes a Day to Ease Aches All Over

Kathryn Ross-Nash
and the editors of Prevention

Contents

Pain-Free Movement Starts Here

▶ **Can you recall** a moment when pain caught you off guard during a task you've done a million times? Maybe your legs unexpectedly ached as you got up from sitting on the floor. Or your back tensed as you reached to grab a glass from a high shelf. These situations can feel like a turning point—the end of an era of easy movement and the beginning of the age of aches, pains, and limitations.

But it doesn't have to be that way. As a physical therapist and Pilates instructor, I've seen people go from struggling with limited mobility to effortlessly doing the things they love once more. The solution doesn't always have to be expensive recovery devices or surgery. In many instances, you can solve your pain problem with something much simpler: stretching.

All stretching is beneficial, but what I've seen work wonders for patients is a plan that mirrors the movements they use in real life—a plan like the one my friend and stretching expert Kathryn Ross-Nash developed for this book.

I've known Kathryn for some 35 years, so I know she's always had a knack for creating programs that meet people where they are—literally! Where are you right now? Sitting at your kitchen table? Lying in bed? This plan has stretches you can do in both of these places to melt away pain. And best of all, this plan takes as little as five minutes a day to do.

This approachability is why I recommend this program to anyone looking for a way to ease pain. Kathryn based this plan around the tasks you already know how to do: pulling a shirt over your head, pushing a grocery cart, walking up stairs. My job as a physical therapist is to help people be able to do all the things they want and need to do. So I can't think of a more effective way to help you move through your day without pain than to teach you stretches that mimic the exact motions you find yourself doing most often. After completing one of Kathryn's plans, you will not only be able to do these everyday activities with less pain, you'll likely be able to do more in general.

With Kathryn's guidance, you'll learn how to align your body for healthy, healing movement (something we could all use after logging countless hours slouched on the couch or hunched over our laptops). But more than that, you'll learn how to move with awareness and intention: how to be present in your body. Paying attention to how your body really feels helps you more precisely identify your pain and work to reduce it. To help you do so, Kathryn has included useful tools like her Active Mobility, Flexibility, and Balance Evaluation; Postural Check-Ins; and advice on alignment. After all, it's hard to manage your pain if you're not moving mindfully. Plus, greater awareness will help you better communicate your pain to a doctor or pain specialist should you ever need to.

I've seen what the power of stretching can do for so many people. It keeps you active and energized, eases pain, and prevents new aches down the road. Anyone can do it. And with this essential guide, I know you're about to enter a new era of pain-free possibility.

Lori Coleman-Brown, P.T.
Director of Education,
Atlas Pilates, Seattle, WA

Introduction

When I was young, I didn't understand pain. Each morning, my feet met the floor and I hit the ground running, moving easily through life.

But one day, everything changed. At age 25, I injured my spine while dancing. I was dropped from a lift and cracked the facet in my spine.

Suddenly, I had to think about the consequences of every movement. While struggling to get out of bed, I learned to take a bodily inventory before moving. My perspective on my body and my relationship with it changed overnight.

I soon learned to adapt and apply my fitness knowledge to my daily life and, later, to the lives of my clients. Each of life's hurdles taught me more, and I was inspired to learn about the importance of body awareness and correct movement. I fit preparing for movement—with movement—into my everyday life, and I'll show you how to do so too.

My name is Kathryn Ross-Nash, and I've spent the last 35-plus years training clients and improving their quality of life when other programs failed. I've done this through correct, clear, and simple movement, and I've trained thousands worldwide to teach my practical method.

Since that first injury, pain has affected me both personally and professionally. As a former professional dancer and a mother of two (with one C-section), I've broken multiple bones, torn muscles, and had dislocated joints. At 58 years old, I cope with several pain-related diagnoses, including illnesses such as ankylosing spondylitis and spondyloarthritis, which are attacking my spine. Fibromyalgia inflames my nerves and causes fatigue and mood issues.

So I understand when clients ask, "What can I do to lessen my pain? How can I feel better?"

You're probably asking that question, too. If you're experiencing serious pain, be sure to consult your doctor before starting any program. But as a Pilates instructor, I have an approach that might help you: I focus on helping clients enjoy mind-body connection benefits through movement. I've worked with professional athletes, physicians, physical therapists, singers, and the severely injured or impaired. Pain knows no limits. But all these success stories share one quality—a training program that met each client where they were and didn't force them into a cookie-cutter mold, a program that accommodated personal needs and goals.

Pilates has been a part of my identity and livelihood for over 45 years because of its healing powers. As you'll see throughout this book, I've selected the best Pilates-inspired stretches to ease pain no matter what aches you may have.

In this book, we will explore a program customized to you. We'll go step-by-step, at your pace, with understandable and digestible exercises you'll want to do. Many exercises are now second nature to me, and I know they can be for you, too.

I'll lead you along, using what I've learned. Every morning before I get out of bed, I warm up, stretch, and prepare to place my feet on the floor. Think about your cat or dog. Does your pet just jump out of bed and dash around the house? Not unless the doorbell rings! No, your companion animal usually stretches from legs to spine—and feels good doing it. Animals prepare for movement, and so should you.

These movements can be free of frustration, strain, and pain and won't feel overwhelming or time-consuming. There's no need to run to the gym, buy expensive equipment, or work out for extended periods. You'll stretch in the privacy of your own home, incorporating movements into everyday life.

Pain robs us of the joy in life—it takes our freedom and makes our world smaller. So I encourage you to exercise to improve your life, not punish your body. Mindset is imperative. I often hear the dread in the voices of people trying to convince themselves to kick off a program or return to the gym. But stretching gives a return to life, freedom, and joyful experiences. When I open my eyes in the morning, I think, "How lucky I am! I have these few minutes to give myself the gift of movement."

Movement can change lives. I see it every day. I look forward to sharing these effective and achievable 28-day programs with you, with some taking as little as five minutes per day. You've already taken the first step if you're reading this. Fantastic! Now let us move and heal!

Kathryn Ross-Nash

▶ **Pain is real, but it doesn't have to be permanent. Recent studies have shown that home-based stretching programs can decrease pain and increase mobility.**

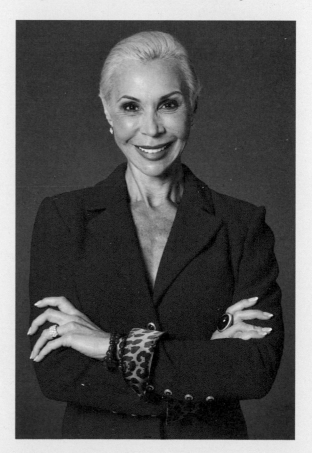

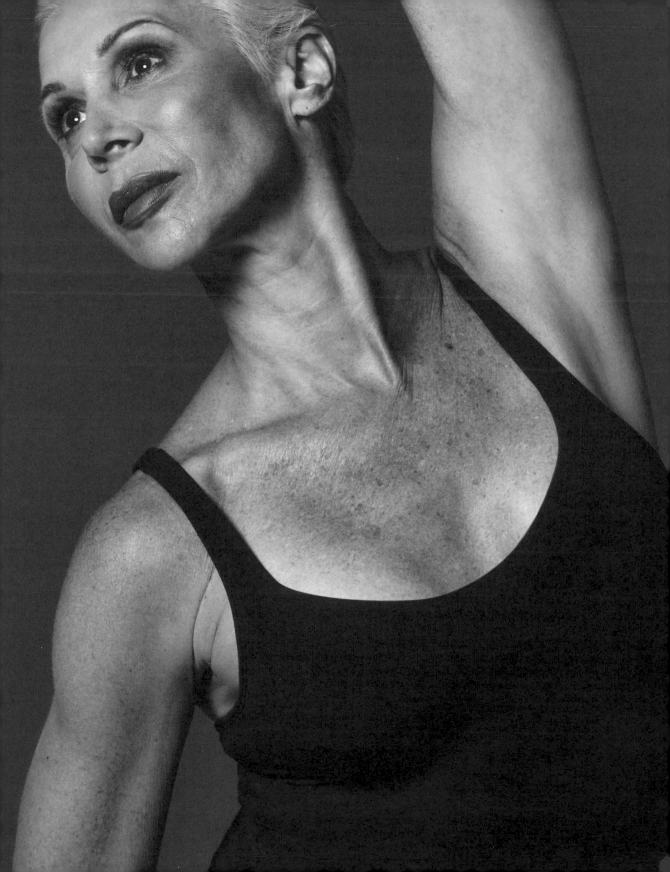

CHAPTER 01

A Practical Pain Solution

If you're reading this book, you've likely been struggling with pain. Perhaps your back has been bothering you, or you seem to wake up with the same kink in your neck every single morning. If that's you, you might find the thought of committing to any type of physical activity daunting. That's understandable. When you're in pain, it can often seem like your best bet is to simply stay put.

But stretching, particularly the kind we'll cover in this book, can help ease the aches you're currently experiencing and prevent new pains. And unlike other forms of exercise that require you to dive right into the deep end, stretching can be done gradually and at your own pace. Most importantly, it just feels great.

Before starting the 28-day plan, familiarize yourself with the fundamentals—why and how stretching works, and how to approach this program from a holistic perspective. If doubts and procrastination crop up as you follow the 28-day plan, revisit this chapter as a reminder of why stretching is such a powerful tool for healing. I hope you'll feel reinspired. Here are four things to know about stretching and how it can improve your life.

STRETCHING EASES EXISTING PAINS AND PREVENTS NEW ONES.

Stretching not only feels good—it does your body good, while also relieving pain. The physical benefits are numerous. Stretching can improve short- and long-term balance and help with medical conditions like degenerative joint disease (osteoarthritis) and frozen shoulder. It also boosts your health by upping oxygen levels, increasing blood flow, and delivering nutrients to your muscles. A good stretch may even reduce arterial stiffening—a hardening of the arteries that occurs with aging—lessening the effort your heart exerts to pump blood through your body. It can also help your heart beat at more regular intervals and improve your resting heart rate. In a nutshell, stretching helps your body function at its best.

So what happens if you don't stretch? Your joints become rigid and more prone to injury. You've probably experienced this in the past—for example, have you ever stepped out of bed too quickly in the morning and felt tightness? Stretching before you place your feet on the floor may offer a very different (and less painful!) morning. Plus, skipping that regular morning stretch session can leave you feeling all wound up and more prone to falls.

A sedentary lifestyle combined with infrequent stretching increases the risk of falling and/or losing real-world functional ability and balance. Every year, 36 million falls happen among adults aged 65 and older, and fall injuries hospitalize more than 950,000 older adults. Falls frequently cause broken bones, hip fractures, and brain injuries, among other issues. Even just a little stretching, like the five minutes a day we'll do in this plan, can help improve your balance and prevent future pain.

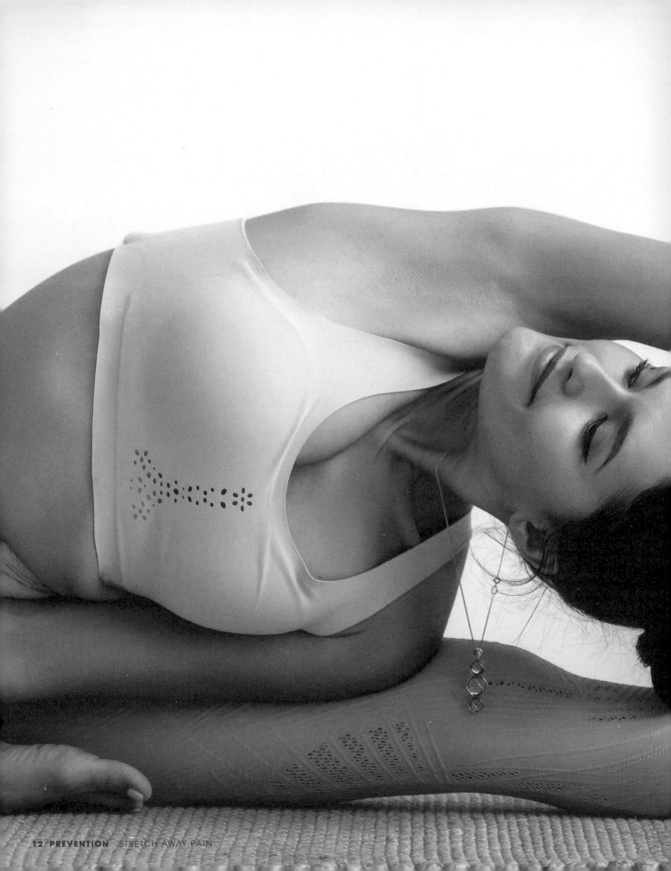

STRETCHING CAN BE ULTRA-EFFICIENT.

There's a lot going on underneath the skin's surface to produce all these positive outcomes. In fact, you may be surprised to learn that a foot stretch reaches all the way to your face!

When you stretch one body part, you get full-body engagement. After all, your muscles, bones, and tendons are all connected—which may be why when you have upper back pain, you'll also end up with a headache later in the day. On top of this, collagen fibers called fascia weave throughout the entire body, creating a network that holds all your joints, muscles, and more in place.

All this interconnectedness means that pain in one area can affect another body part. But it also means you get more bang for your buck when you stretch. If you stretch one muscle series, you can address multiple areas of pain at once.

For this reason, I don't break down stretches into individual body parts, but rather into broader movements. Any stretch in this book reflects the fact that every fiber is interconnected and affected by movement. These exercises were created to address the body as one unit, holistically. In other words, you get more out of every movement in this book—which I know is crucial when everyday tasks like getting out of bed or taking the stairs can trigger pain.

Fast Fact

Long-term flexibility gained when young seems to follow us into adulthood. So even if you haven't touched your toes since high school gym class, you may find you're currently more limber than you think!

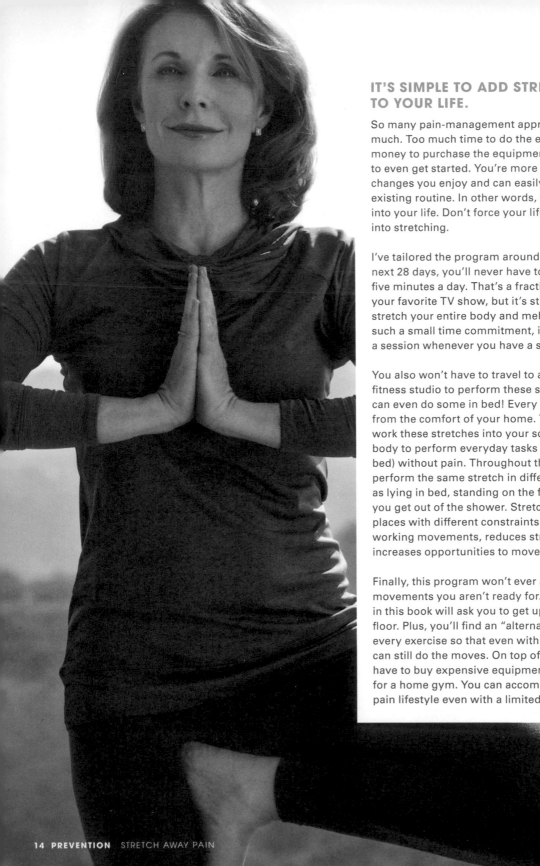

IT'S SIMPLE TO ADD STRETCHING TO YOUR LIFE.

So many pain-management approaches ask too much. Too much time to do the exercises, too much money to purchase the equipment, too much effort to even get started. You're more likely to stick with changes you enjoy and can easily integrate into your existing routine. In other words, stretching should fit into your life. Don't force your life to fit into stretching.

I've tailored the program around this idea. During the next 28 days, you'll never have to stretch more than five minutes a day. That's a fraction of an episode of your favorite TV show, but it's still enough time to stretch your entire body and melt away aches. With such a small time commitment, it's easy to sneak in a session whenever you have a spare moment.

You also won't have to travel to a gym or special fitness studio to perform these stretches. In fact, you can even do some in bed! Every move can be done from the comfort of your home. That lets you easily work these stretches into your schedule to train your body to perform everyday tasks (like getting out of bed) without pain. Throughout the book, I ask you to perform the same stretch in different locations, such as lying in bed, standing on the floor, or right when you get out of the shower. Stretching in different places with different constraints eases daily life's working movements, reduces stress and pain, and increases opportunities to move away from pain.

Finally, this program won't ever ask you to perform movements you aren't ready for. Not one stretch in this book will ask you to get up or down from the floor. Plus, you'll find an "alternative stretch" for every exercise so that even with limited mobility, you can still do the moves. On top of all that, you won't have to buy expensive equipment or carve out room for a home gym. You can accomplish a reduced-pain lifestyle even with a limited space or budget.

STRETCHING MAKES YOUR DAILY LIFE EASIER.

After you learn the stretches in this book, you can "translate" them to functional activities—how to properly reach for an item perched on a high shelf, for example. After all, if a stretch doesn't help you move with less pain in the real world, what good is it? As you develop mental and physical shortcuts, you'll easily solve movement problems.

For example, driving requires the ability to turn and look at a rearview mirror. Using rotation stretches can increase and improve both the range and ease of your upper-body rotation, and the shoulder mobility needed to do so. Or consider the movements needed to crouch down to clean an awkward place, such as under the kitchen table. Stretches like extended cat and cat and cow (pages 134 and 135) help you complete these tasks without pain.

I created the book's exercises to build functional movement, to improve your flexibility with each stretch—and to help you find freedom through flexibility. Here are a few ways to apply some of the book's exercises to decrease pain in your daily life.

Do Everyday Tasks with Less Pain

Reaching an object on a higher shelf	**BED STRETCHES** Side-to-Side Stretches (p. 81)
Walking up stairs	**BED STRETCHES** Single-Knee Hugs (p. 83)
Walking on flat ground	**SEATED CHAIR STRETCHES** Four Parts of the Foot (p. 121)
Removing a shirt by pulling it overhead	**BED STRETCHES** Full-Body Stretch with Arm Arcs (p. 74)
Getting in and out of a car or bathtub	**BED STRETCHES** Windshield Wipers (p. 89)
Putting on and taking off coats and jackets	**BED STRETCHES** Windshield Wipers (p. 89) and Single-Leg Twists (p. 88)

As I mentioned earlier, one of the most important things you can do to prevent pain is to improve your balance. That's why I've also included stretches to help you achieve and maintain flexibility and balance for independent everyday life. Many factors contribute to balance loss, and this loss leads to increased falls and injuries. I've witnessed huge decreases in balance ability when a client comes to me after being sedentary for an extended period.

Daily life offers endless hidden gems of movement opportunities, moments that let you stretch and enjoy the activities of daily life. As you go about your day, identify the movements you often repeat. Recognizing patterns helps you develop a cognitive map of your environment and provides more movement awareness. Perhaps you'll find you often repeat the same arm-raised movement of pulling a shirt overhead (maybe when you're clapping your hands overhead at a football game or dancing at a concert). Then you might make the full-body stretch on page 94 part of your daily routine even after completing the 28-day plan.

Always be on the lookout for these little treasures. I'm surprised at how many places I've found the movements listed in this book. You can even use them as a cue to stretch! Adding stretches to daily activities won't fatigue and tighten your body, but instead will give you an added burst of pain relief. You'll likely find that everyday tasks become a little easier and more enjoyable.

Fast Fact

Studies show that a person's ability to stand on one leg for 10 seconds can determine overall health and longevity.

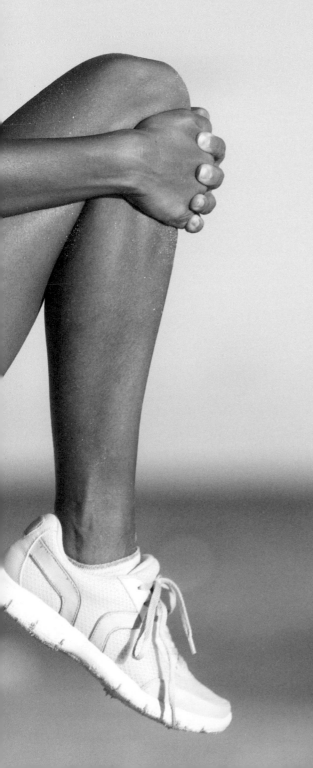

Use Your Brain to Soothe Pain

The more stressed you are, the more pain you feel. Mindfulness techniques can dial down that tension and prevent hurt. You can mix and match the techniques below; just aim for two or three 5-minute sessions a day.

CONDUCT A BODY SCAN

Lie down and bring your attention to your toes. Acknowledge all sensations, painful or pleasant, without judgment, then breathe into them. Continue this for your whole body, up to the top of your head.

BREATHE DEEPLY

Sitting or lying down, place one hand on your abdomen and the other on your chest. Inhale slowly through your nose and into your belly. Pause a few seconds, then exhale slowly through your mouth. Repeat until you feel calmer.

MEDITATE

Sit comfortably and bring your awareness to the present moment. Notice what's happening, physically and emotionally, right now—not in the future or past. Mind strays? Gently bring it back.

Three Steps for Stretching Success

What makes stretching such a practical solution to pain is how little you need to get started: just yourself and a positive mindset! Here are three strategies to keep your motivation high for the next 28 days.

1 FIND YOUR ANGLE

Seek your personal, positive motivation by considering what you'll gain. What makes you commit? What excites you? What will you get out of this experience? I love to use mantras to keep my motivation in focus. Mantras break negative thought cycles and support us. The word "mantra" originates from Sanskrit, which combines the root words "manas," meaning to think and "tra," meaning vehicle. Using a mantra transports us to our goals. A mantra can be a repeatable sound, a thought, or a word to increase experiential presence and keep you focused and connected. I translate mantra as connecting your body to your mind. Create your own mantra or try one of my personal favorites on page 20.

2 MAKE A PLAN

Identify when you will stretch each day and write it on your calendar. Treat it like an appointment with yourself. Consistency creates success. I schedule my stretches for the same time each day and before I begin my other commitments. Otherwise, it's too easy for other routines, tasks, and chores to swallow my time. Prioritize your well-being by putting movement on your to-do list—and even use your phone to set reminders to stretch.

With any new endeavor, there may be moments along the way when you feel like quitting, so plan for them. We all have reasons we don't exercise, which can stymie our progress—or maybe we just avoid getting started. Here are four very common rationalizations you might come up with, and how to reframe the obstacle into an opportunity.

PROBLEM: LACK OF TIME
SOLUTION: This book asks for just five minutes daily, often incorporated into your daily routine, rather than added to an already-busy day. Stretch in your bed before you rise or after your morning shower. Integrate stretches into your everyday activities.

PROBLEM: TOO DIFFICULT
SOLUTION: You won't be able to perform all exercises immediately. But we all learn our alphabet before we read. Working out follows the same principles. Begin with your movement ABCs, and soon, you'll be reading *Romeo and Juliet.*

PROBLEM: FEAR OF FAILURE
SOLUTION: Starting anything is difficult and sometimes even a little scary. If you've missed or skipped a few days, that's okay—just go back to the beginning and restart the program with the first step of day one. It might not be easy to take that first step, but this book will prepare you to take that initial movement over and over.

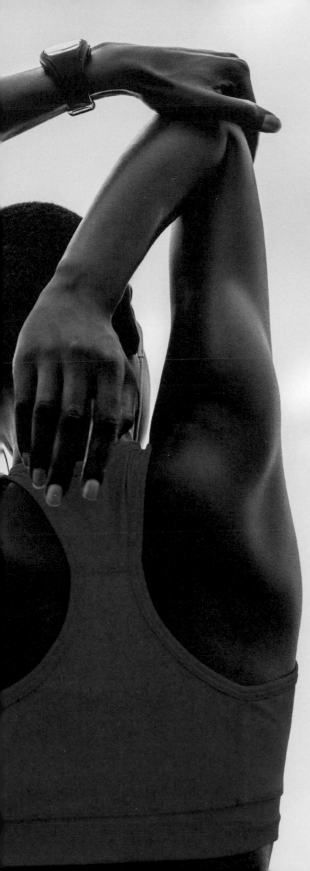

PROBLEM: NO MOTIVATION

SOLUTION: Encourage accountability by asking a friend or family member to stretch with you for the next 28 days, or otherwise check in. This works! Many clients have asked me to text and check that they did the work. Such support from friends and family can offer beneficial outcomes when setting a goal to prioritize well-being.

3 BEGIN WHERE YOU ARE

This program is about easing your aches and pains, so listen to your body and don't push to do something you're not ready for. Take the Active Mobility, Flexibility, and Balance Evaluation on page 28 before moving on to the 28-day plan. Your results will inform what stretches you should start with. Watch how stretching impacts your tests over time, and see if easier movement helps build pain prevention and relief.

When you're ready to kick off the program, begin slowly, with no more than 15 minutes a day. Even if you think you can do more, don't try it. You're more likely to continue training if you stick to 15 minutes daily and leave your body craving more versus doing more, overextending yourself, and dreading stretches. These short training sessions will boost your energy and sharpen your focus.

Feel free to do these stretching plans with any other pain-free exercise you enjoy, like walking or swimming. Every day, we'll add movements to your routine. But no rush—only tack those on if you feel ready. After 28 days, modify or adjust the program based on what worked best for you.

A Motivating Mantra

▶ FOCUS

Focus brings your attention to and connects you to where your body is at, in exactly this moment. The past may cause sadness, while the future may inspire anxiety. With intention, you enter this moment—all you have and where we begin.

▶ FEEL

Feel each movement as you stretch. Feel your lungs expand with each breath, stretching your rib cage and spine. Feel muscles happily moving from toe-tip to fingertip. Feel the circulation moving through your body.

▶ FUNCTION

Movement improves daily life functions and tasks. Real-life actions inspired these stretches, all formulated and developed to meet your personal needs.

▶ FREEDOM

Imagine the freedom to move with less pain. Your dedication will impact your outcomes. The more effort you put into the program (and yourself), the more you'll get out of it. Movement heals.

For this book, I created the Four Fs mantra above to strengthen your motivation and grounding. Say "Focus. Feel. Function. Freedom." upon waking up and whenever you need a boost of encouragement. I use this mantra to begin my day and whenever I need inspiration.

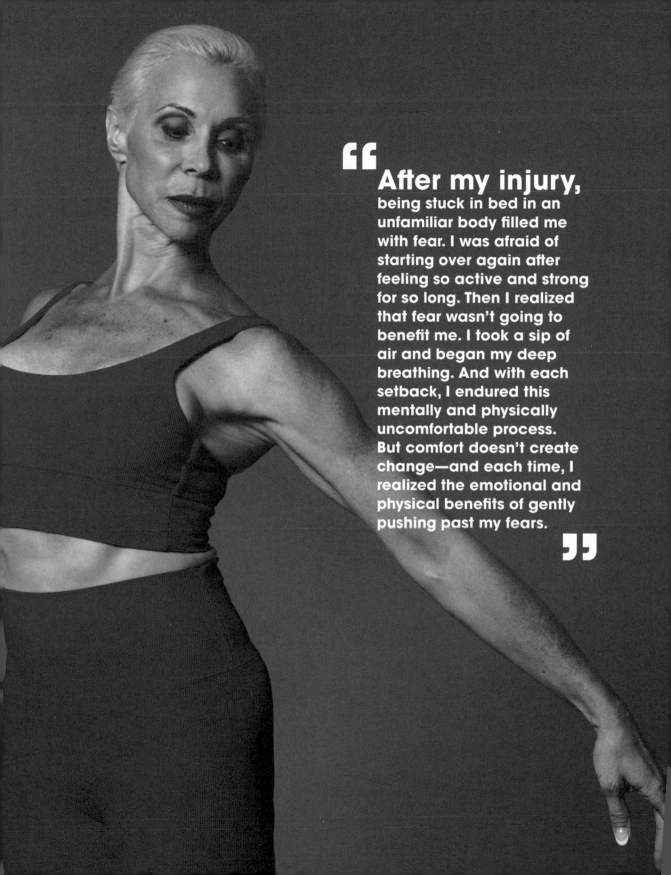

" After my injury, being stuck in bed in an unfamiliar body filled me with fear. I was afraid of starting over again after feeling so active and strong for so long. Then I realized that fear wasn't going to benefit me. I took a sip of air and began my deep breathing. And with each setback, I endured this mentally and physically uncomfortable process. But comfort doesn't create change—and each time, I realized the emotional and physical benefits of gently pushing past my fears. **"**

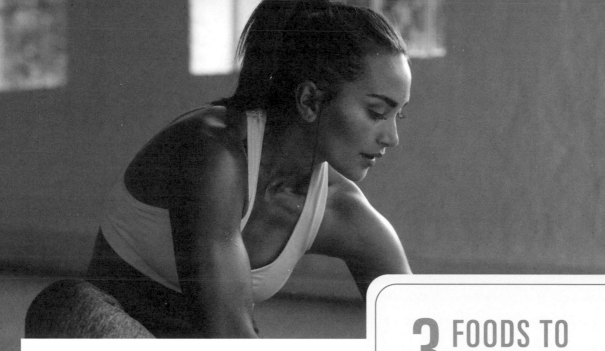

▶ Stretching FAQs

Here are all the questions I get asked—with answers!

Q: WHAT'S THE RELATIONSHIP BETWEEN STRETCHING AND PAIN?

A: As you age, your body becomes increasingly stiff as blood flow decreases, leading to less well-lubricated muscles and joints. Stretching your body is like running your car's engine regularly. After all, if your car sits for months, what happens? It doesn't start. Daily stretching keeps your motor running and prevents stiffened joints, which helps avoid painful joints.

Q: HOW DOES STRETCHING PREVENT PAIN?

A: Stretching improves joint function and balance, lowering your risk of injury and increasing your coordination. Stretching increases flexibility and strength, enabling you to move freely through your daily life. This usually means that you have better dexterity and balance, and increased range of motion. For example, daily shoulder rolls may lessen the tension in your neck, so you can more easily check your blind spot with a head turn while driving.

3 FOODS TO FIGHT ACHES

Natural remedies have been used to soothe pain for centuries. Try adding these to your diet.

FISH OIL
Studies show that the fatty acids in fish oil can help people with morning stiffness, painful joints, and lack of strength in their hands.

TURMERIC
Curcumin, the yellow compound that's found in turmeric, is being studied as a potential way to prevent or help treat arthritis pain.

CHAMOMILE TEA
Compounds in the chamomile flower can lower inflammation, calm your entire nervous system, and help lull you to sleep.

Q: HOW DOES STRETCHING RELIEVE PAIN?

A: Stretching increases pain tolerance and increases range of motion and healing circulation in the painful area, which relaxes tight muscles and relieves stress. As a bonus, stretching boosts your mood and develops stronger muscles to prevent future pain.

Q: HOW CAN I TELL IF I'M PERFORMING THE STRETCH CORRECTLY?

A: Listen to your body and learn its signals for pain. You should feel some "good" pain, or mild discomfort, when stretching. This pain is dull, never sharp, and doesn't increase as you move. "Bad" pain is sharp. Consider it a red light! It means you should stop immediately.

Q: WHY DO YOU NEED TO STRETCH YOUR ENTIRE BODY, NOT JUST THE PAINFUL BODY PART?

A: If your lower back is bugging you, you may be tempted to go directly to a stretch focused on the back and ignore the rest. But only working one body part leaves the rest of you susceptible to pain. Plus, as mentioned earlier, everything in your body is interconnected. Ever stub your toe and have your shoulders shoot up to your ears? Localized pain—whether chronic or acute—can affect the whole body. Stretching holistically also offers all the benefits of lowering injury risk, increasing your flexibility and strength, and enabling more unrestricted movement through daily life.

Q: WHAT'S THE DIFFERENCE BETWEEN CHRONIC AND ACUTE PAIN?

A: Chronic pain is a pain you've had for at least three to six months and takes a serious mental and physical toll. For example, chronic pain is usually associated with health issues such as arthritis, spinal conditions, fibromyalgia, and many other lasting health conditions. The 28-day plan in this book will help you work through such pains. On the other hand, sometimes the pain you're experiencing sneaks up on you out of the blue, like a back ache from sleeping on a pull-out couch. This is acute pain. Often, acute pain is directly linked to something you did, like sleeping on that unsupportive sofa, and begins to diminish when you stop doing that thing, like when you go back to dozing on your own bed. But, of course, life happens. When it does, try these stretches to soothe whatever unexpected ache creeps up.

Feel Better Fast

Acute Pain	Stretches
You have a kink in your neck after sleeping wrong	**BED STRETCHES** Shoulder Drops (p. 76) **POST-SHOWER STRETCHES** Shoulder Rolls (p. 96)
Your back is sore from lifting a heavy box	**BED STRETCHES** Single-Knee Hugs (p. 83)
Your legs are painfully stiff after sitting for too long	**BED STRETCHES** Ankle Stretch (p. 79) Hamstring Stretch (p. 87) Climb a Tree (p. 86)
Your shoulders ache from driving in traffic	**BED STRETCHES** Shoulder Drops (p. 76) Roll-Up Back Stretch (p. 84) **POST-SHOWER STRETCHES** Shoulder Rolls (p. 96)
Your hands hurt from hours spent typing	**BED STRETCHES** Flex, Extend, and Circles (p. 77)
Your back hurts from golfing	**BED STRETCHES** Windshield Wipers (p. 89) Single-Leg Twists (p. 88) **SEATED CHAIR STRETCHES** Towel Twist (p. 132) Hand Clasp Arm and Shoulder Stretch (p. 133)
You're stressed and feel like you need to take a deep breath	**BREATHWORK** Deep Breathing (p. 71) Progressive Breathing (p. 70)

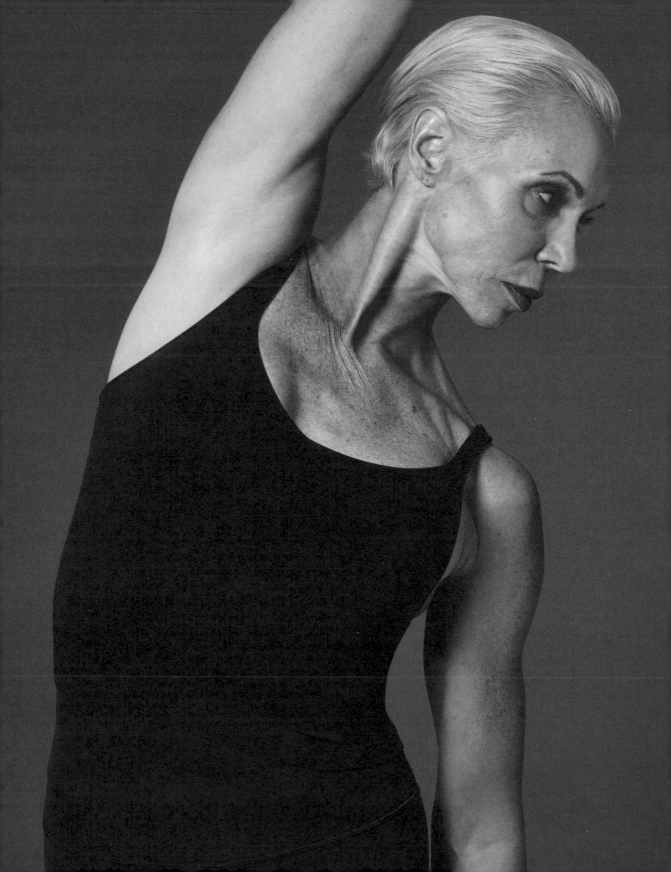

CHAPTER 02

Find Your Starting Point

When it comes to stretching, you have to learn what works for your unique needs. We all begin at different points, with different types and levels of pain. Wherever you're starting from, you're in the perfect place to begin stretching to ease your aches. Later in this book you'll see I've included dozens of stretches for all types of pain, plus an alternative stretch for each exercise. Every stretch in this book will do wonders for your mobility, so you can't go wrong no matter which exercise you pick.

To help you feel more comfortable from the outset, I've developed a total-body stretching evaluation that will help you determine what stretches to start with. Selecting the right stretches helps you better address your unique needs, and it maintains motivation. Starting small, perhaps below the point you think you're ready for, will make every step forward feel like a win (because it is!). It may be tempting to dive straight into the deep end, but a gradual approach will serve you best in the long run.

As you complete this evaluation, remember: There are no "wrong" answers to the questions on the following pages. Be honest with yourself and don't stretch to the point of "bad" pain. As you complete this evaluation starting on page 28, don't forget to follow the suggestions at the end of the chapter. Be sure to flip back to this section throughout the 28-day program to reflect on where you started and celebrate just how far you've come!

Before You Begin

Before performing your evaluation or any of the stretches throughout the program, follow these guidelines.

▶ **SEE YOUR DOC.**

Always consult a medical professional before beginning this or any other movement-based activity. If you're unsure if you should do a certain exercise, don't do it, especially if you have medical contraindications.

▶ **DO A LITTLE PREP WORK.**

Get any clothing and props ready to go before training to avoid procrastination and to encourage new habits. I have a dedicated place for my workouts, a little place of peace. I suggest setting up for the next day right after completing the day's stretches and keeping your space neat, organized, and welcoming!

▶ DRESS FOR SUCCESS—AND COMFORT.

Support the body parts that need support and allow the rest to breathe. I usually wear a sports bra, a T-shirt, and leggings or sweatpants. If you're moving in cooler weather, wear something warmer, but avoid tight attire or anything that inhibits movement.

▶ READ EACH EXERCISE LIKE A RECIPE.

Read movement instructions three times before attempting the movement for the first time. On the following days, read instructions twice until you're familiar with the instructions. Nothing is worse than forgetting a step and ending up undercooked!

▶ UNDERSTAND PROPER ALIGNMENT.

This one's especially important. With everyday life often demanding we crane our necks to look at laptop screens and smartphones, it's easy to forget about posture. You might not realize you're rounding your back and jutting your neck out to read your texts, but over time poor posture can lead to health issues and put stress on your joints and spine.

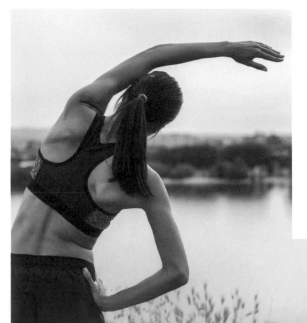

Proper posture or alignment is critical to performing the book's stretches. Your muscles and joints work most efficiently when properly aligned. It helps create optimal force when needed to complete a movement or task and reduces force where we don't want it, decreasing the risk of injury. In short, you'll get the biggest benefits from each move with the least strain on your body.

So what does being in alignment look like? It's when your head, shoulders, spine, hips, knees, ankles, and feet line up. Imagine a line that runs through the center of each joint where they connect. In many cases, it's easier to identify good posture by what it isn't. Be mindful of these negative postural habits:

- **Slumping forward**
- **Arching your lower back**
- **Pressing your hips forward**
- **Rounding your upper back**
- **Twisting your hips or shoulders**
- **Shortening one side of your waist**

Read the exercise's important cues focused on alignment. A picture is worth a thousand words, so use the accompanying photos to further understand alignment requirements. The white arrows in each photo demonstrate alignment clarity and are key to improving your results.

- **When you're in alignment, a stretch may be uncomfortable but not painful. You may be stretching parts that typically avoid being stretched.**

- **If your body is out of alignment, you won't stretch the specific muscles necessary, as your body tends to take the path of least resistance and stretch what isn't tight.**

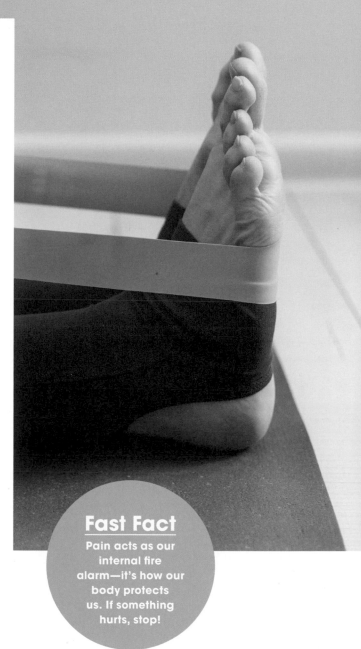

▶ DISTINGUISH "GOOD" PAIN FROM "BAD" PAIN.

A "good pain" may feel more like tightness or stiffness as you begin a stretch, which gently increases healing circulation and alleviates pain in stiff areas. But sharp or burning pain warns that something is wrong—avoid that pain as much as possible. If a movement is painful, it is not for you. If your knee hurts, don't bend it to the point of sharp pain. If it hurts to turn your head to the right, focus on shoulder drops or rolls to stretch the neck muscles without moving the neck itself.

- **Respect your internal cues. Pain is just one of them. Other warning signs that are telling you to pause or stop include feeling dizzy, flushed, or exhausted. You may be pushing too much or have an underlying issue that needs to be addressed.**

- **Be careful not to overstretch. It can cause micro-trauma or tears in the muscles or connective tissue and result in an injury, such as a strain or sprain. Feeling sore the day after stretching or experiencing a sharp or stabbing pain means that you're stretching your muscles beyond their capacity for flexibility. When in doubt, go slowly.**

- **When doing these tests, don't push too hard—I recommend 70% of your potential. Think of 70% as work that's somewhere in the middle, between the most you can push a stretch and the least you can push a stretch. Pushing to the maximum movement can cause injury—but progress doesn't occur if you're only using minimum effort. Prioritize the quality of movement over the quantity of movement. The same is true for repetitions, for which I offer only a suggested number. Complete what you can do cleanly, with clarity and control.**

Fast Fact

Pain acts as our internal fire alarm—it's how our body protects us. If something hurts, stop!

Active Mobility, Flexibility, and Balance Evaluation

To complete the evaluation, you will need a stopwatch and a ruler. Follow the instructions, and after you've done each exercise, circle the letter (A, B, C, or D) that applies to you.

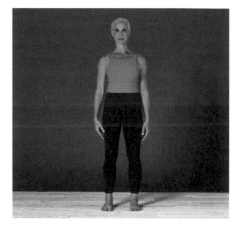

1. LUNG CAPACITY TEST

Stand with your legs sit-bone-width apart and parallel, feet and knees facing forward, and arms at your sides. Pretend you're putting on a pair of tight jeans and pull in your tummy.

MOVEMENT

1. Inhale as fully and as deeply as you can.
2. Hold your breath. Count or time how many seconds you can hold it.
3. Exhale.

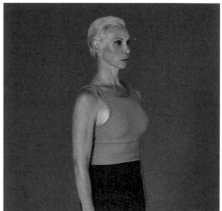

HOW LONG WERE YOU ABLE TO HOLD YOUR BREATH?

A. 90 seconds
B. 60 seconds
C. 30 seconds
D. Less than 30 seconds

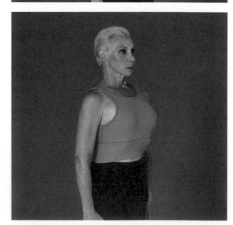

2. NECK MOBILITY AND FLEXIBILITY TEST

Stand with your legs sit-bone-width apart and parallel, feet and knees facing forward, and arms at your sides. Zip up those tight jeans!

MOVEMENT

1. Make a fist with your right hand and place it, thumb down, on your right shoulder.
2. Tip your head to reach your right ear toward your right shoulder.
3. Perform the same move on the other side.

HOW CLOSE TO BOTH SHOULDERS WERE YOU ABLE TO TIP YOUR HEAD?

A. Your ear touches the hand on both sides.
B. Your ear touches the hand on one side, but it hurts or is difficult to tip your head on the other.
C. Your ear hovers near the hand on both sides.
D. It hurts to tip your head on both sides.

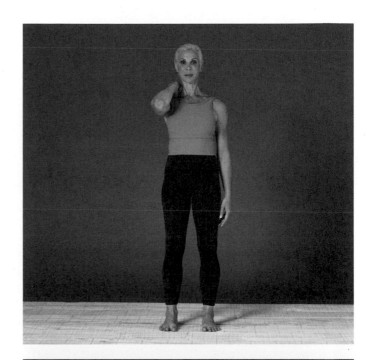

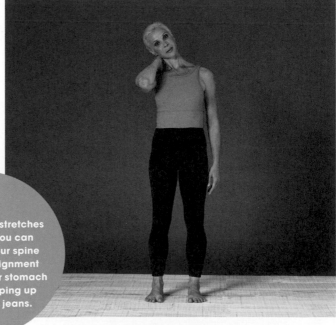

Tip

For many of the stretches in this book, you can help protect your spine and support alignment by pulling in your stomach as if you're zipping up a tight pair of jeans.

3. FORWARD STRETCH ABILITY TEST

Sit on a sturdy chair. Place both feet flat on the floor, sit-bone-width apart and parallel. Keep the ball of each foot in line with its heel, knee, and hip. Keep the arch of the foot lifted by pressing your big toe and heel into the floor and rotating your foot to its outer edge.

MOVEMENT

1. Extend one leg forward and in line with its hip. Keep your leg in line with your hip and keep the knee and the toes pointed to the ceiling. Don't overextend the knee.
2. Flex the foot so that the toes point upward.
3. With fingers extended, reach both hands toward your flexed toes. Keep your shoulders and hips parallel to each other.
4. Measure how far down your leg you can reach. Repeat on the second side.

HOW FAR CAN YOU STRETCH?

A. You can reach your toes or beyond with a straight leg.
B. You can reach your shin.
C. You can reach your knee.
D. You experience discomfort and need to bend your leg.

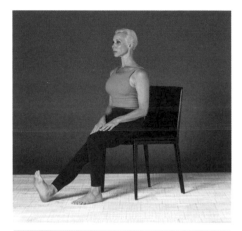

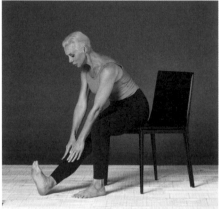

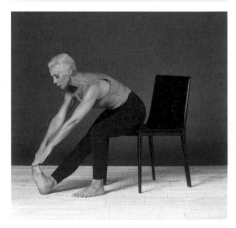

4. ROTATION ABILITY TEST

Sit on a sturdy chair. Place both feet flat on the floor, sit-bone-width apart and parallel.

MOVEMENT

1. Lift your arms in front of you at shoulder height. Keeping your arms at shoulder height, bend your elbows and stack your forearms, fingertip to elbow, with your right arm on top. Shoulders and forearms are parallel.
2. Inhale and pull your stomach in to protect your spine. Feel as if a corset is around your waist. Remember to breathe.
3. Without moving from the hips down, rotate to the left, letting your gaze follow your left elbow. Lift your ribs off the hips, and don't arch your lower back. Return to center.
4. Without moving from the hips down, rotate to the right. Your gaze should follow your right elbow. Return to center.
5. Repeat steps 2 through 4, this time with your left arm on top.

HOW FAR CAN YOU TURN?

A. Through the shoulders, rib cage, and waist to see behind you.
B. Through the shoulders and rib cage to see halfway behind you.
C. Through the shoulders to see one-quarter of the way behind you.
D. You can't. You have pain when you rotate or turn your head; you must move your hips and pelvis or experience difficulty seeing past your shoulder.

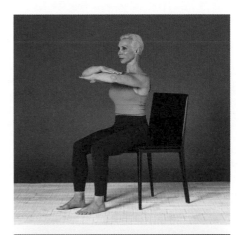

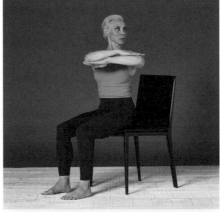

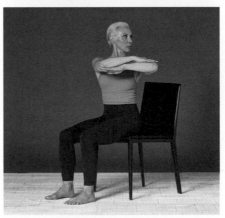

5. SHOULDER AND UPPER BACK MOBILITY AND FLEXIBILITY TEST

Stand with your back to a wall. Legs are sit-bone-width apart and parallel, feet and knees facing forward. Zip up those tight jeans! Press your torso against the wall.

MOVEMENT

1. Walk your feet 6 to 8 inches in front of you.
2. Soften your knees so your back is flush with the wall. Your hips, knees, second toes, and center of your heels are in alignment with each other.
3. On a deep inhalation through your nose, lift your arms to shoulder height and align with your shoulders. Your palms should face down, with your arms straight but not locked.
4. Continue to inhale and reach your arms overhead toward the wall. Palms face forward.

HOW FAR DO YOUR ARMS REACH?

A. The backs of your hands touch the wall behind you.
B. Your arms line up with your ears or face.
C. Your arms stop at the midpoint between your shoulders and your ears.
D. It hurts to attempt to lift your arms above your shoulders.

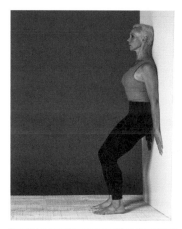

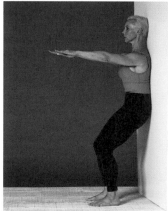

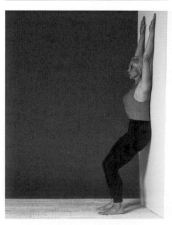

6. SHOULDER AND SIDES MOBILITY AND FLEXIBILITY TEST

Stand against the wall with your legs sit-bone-width apart and parallel, feet and knees facing forward, arms by your sides. Zip up those tight jeans!

MOVEMENT

1. On a deep inhalation through your nose, lift your right arm to shoulder height in front of you and in line with your shoulders. Your palm faces down, and your arm is straight but not locked.
2. Continue to inhale and reach your right arm up and toward the wall. Palm faces forward.
3. Place your left hand on your left side. Bend to the left and slide your left hand down along the left side of your body.
4. Return to upright and switch your arm positions.
5. Slide your right hand down your right leg.

HOW FAR DOES THE HAND THAT'S SLIDING ALONG THE SIDE OF YOUR BODY REACH?

A. Past your knee on both sides.
B. To your knee on both sides.
C. To your mid-thigh on both sides.
D. It hurts to side bend on one or both sides.

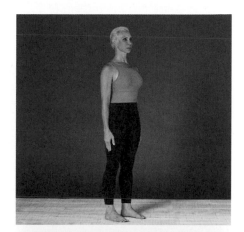

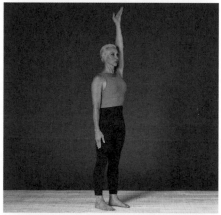

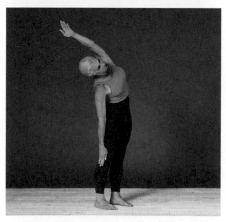

7. STANDING BALANCE TEST

Stand with legs together and parallel, feet pointing forward. Stand with your shoulders over your hips and your weight slightly forward, with 60% of your weight on the balls of your feet. Don't overextend your knees, and keep your hips over your heels. Put your arms down by your sides with palms toward your legs.

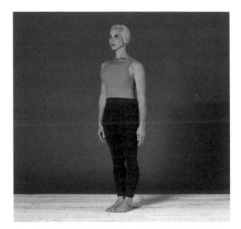

Note: Be sure to execute this in a safe area in case you lose your balance. You may not find your balance right away. Allow yourself a few tries to find your balance. Choosing a focal point will also help.

MOVEMENT

1. Inhale and pull the stomach in to protect the spine. It should feel as if a corset is around your waist. Remember to breathe.
2. Choose a focal point.
3. Without lifting your hip, lift one leg with a bent knee.
4. Count or time how long you can hold your leg up.
5. Place the foot down and repeat on the other side.

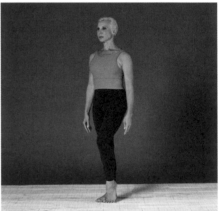

HOW LONG CAN YOU HOLD YOUR LEG UP?

A. Can hold balance 15 seconds or more.
B. Can hold balance 10 seconds.
C. Can hold balance 5 seconds.
D. Unable to balance on one leg.

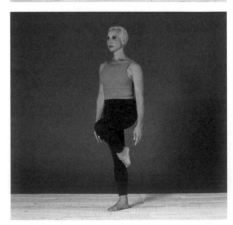

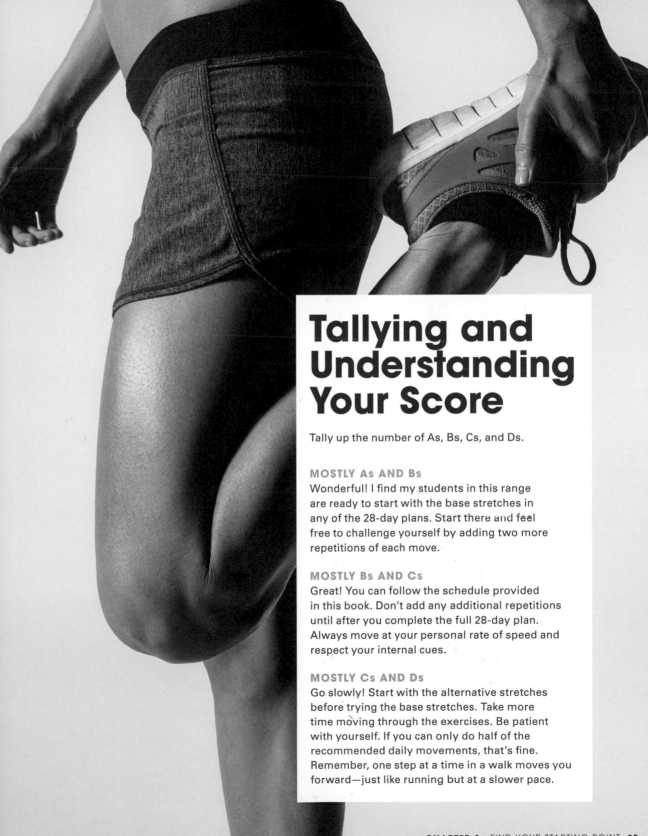

Tallying and Understanding Your Score

Tally up the number of As, Bs, Cs, and Ds.

MOSTLY As AND Bs

Wonderful! I find my students in this range are ready to start with the base stretches in any of the 28-day plans. Start there and feel free to challenge yourself by adding two more repetitions of each move.

MOSTLY Bs AND Cs

Great! You can follow the schedule provided in this book. Don't add any additional repetitions until after you complete the full 28-day plan. Always move at your personal rate of speed and respect your internal cues.

MOSTLY Cs AND Ds

Go slowly! Start with the alternative stretches before trying the base stretches. Take more time moving through the exercises. Be patient with yourself. If you can only do half of the recommended daily movements, that's fine. Remember, one step at a time in a walk moves you forward—just like running but at a slower pace.

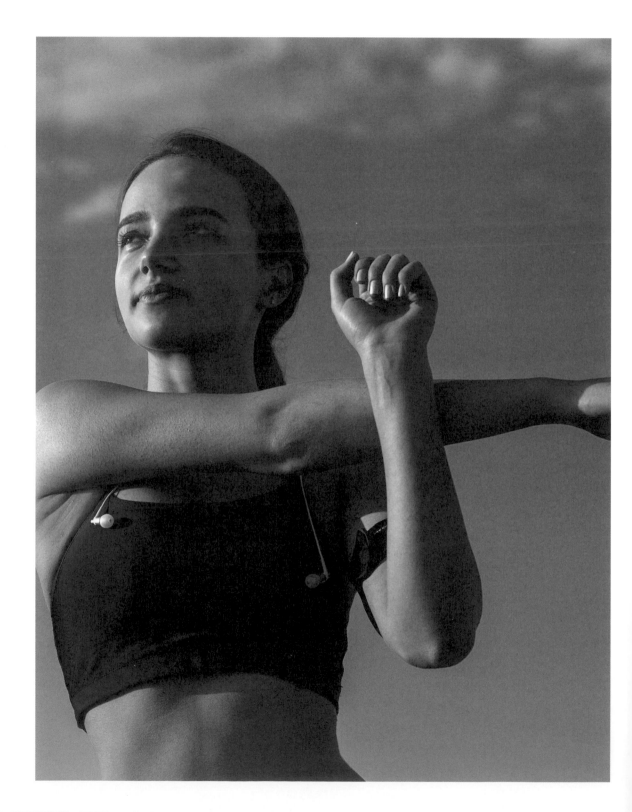

Improve Your Scores

You'll naturally increase your mobility, flexibility, and balance by completing the 28-day program, but if you'd like to home in on a specific area, follow the suggestions in this chart.

If you scored a C or a D on the test, focus on the alternative stretches.
If you scored an A or B, try the base version of the stretches.

Area	Stretches
Lung Capacity Test	**BED STRETCHES** Progressive Breathing (p. 70) **ALTERNATIVE:** Deep Breathing (p. 71) Full-Body Stretch with Arm Arcs (p. 74) **ALTERNATIVE:** Two-Way Stretch (p. 75) **SEATED STRETCHES** Progressive Breathing (p. 70) **ALTERNATIVE:** Deep Breathing (p. 71) Full-Body Stretch with Arm Arcs (p. 114) **ALTERNATIVE:** Two-Way Stretch (p. 115) **WALL STRETCHES** Progressive Breathing (p. 70) **ALTERNATIVE:** Deep Breathing (p. 71)
Neck Mobility and Flexibility Test	**BED STRETCHES** Shoulder Drops (p. 76) **ALTERNATIVE:** Flex, Extend, and Circle (p. 77) **POST-SHOWER STRETCHES** Shoulder Rolls (p. 96) **ALTERNATIVE:** Alternating Arm Arcs (p. 97) **SEATED STRETCHES** Ear and Shoulder Taps (p. 116) **ALTERNATIVE:** Yes and No (p. 117) Extended Cat (p. 134) **ALTERNATIVE:** Cat and Cow (p. 135)

Forward-Stretch Ability Test	**BED STRETCHES** Double-Knee Hug (p. 82) **ALTERNATIVE:** Single-Knee Hug (p. 83) Roll-Up Back Stretch (p. 84) **ALTERNATIVE:** Knee Circle Hug (p. 85) **POST-SHOWER STRETCHES** The Roll Down (p. 104) **ALTERNATIVE:** Standing Upper Back Stretch (p. 105) **SEATED STRETCHES** Forward Stretch Seated with Towel with Twist (p. 124) **ALTERNATIVE:** Forward Stretch Seated with Towel (p. 125) Hamstring Stretch with Towel (p. 126) **ALTERNATIVE:** Single-Knee Lifts with Towel (p. 127)
Rotation Ability Test	**BED STRETCHES** Single-Leg Twists (p. 88) **ALTERNATIVE:** Windshield Wipers (p. 89) **POST-SHOWER STRETCHES** Genie Twist (p. 106) **ALTERNATIVE:** Twist with One Hand on the Wall (p. 107) **SEATED STRETCHES** Towel Twist (p. 132) **ALTERNATIVE:** Hand Clasp Arm and Shoulder Stretch (p. 133)
Shoulder and Upper Back Mobility and Flexibility Test	**BED STRETCHES** Full-Body Stretch with Arm Arcs (p. 74) **ALTERNATIVE:** Two-Way Stretch (p. 75) Shoulder Drops (p. 76) **ALTERNATIVE:** Flex, Extend, and Circle (p. 77) **POST-SHOWER STRETCHES** Shoulder Rolls (p. 96) **ALTERNATIVE:** Alternating Arm Arcs (p. 97) **SEATED STRETCHES** Seated Cheerleader Towel Stretch (p. 118) **ALTERNATIVE:** Towel Shoulder Stretch (p. 119)

Shoulder and Sides Mobility and Flexibility Test	**BED STRETCHES** Side Stretch Legs Bent (p. 80) **ALTERNATIVE:** Side-to-Side Stretches (p. 81) Roll-Up Back Stretch (p. 84) **ALTERNATIVE:** Knee Circle Hug (p. 85) **POST-SHOWER STRETCHES** Side Bend (p. 102) **ALTERNATIVE:** Side Stretch (p. 103) **SEATED STRETCHES** Bottoms Up, Down, and Around (p. 128) **ALTERNATIVE:** Bottoms Up and Down (p. 129) Forward Stretch Seated with Towel with Twist (p. 124) **ALTERNATIVE:** Forward Stretch Seated with Towel (p. 125)
Standing Balance Test	**BED STRETCHES** Single-Leg Back Squat (p. 90) **ALTERNATIVE:** Standing Squat (p. 91) **POST-SHOWER STRETCHES** Standing Ankle Circles (p. 100) **ALTERNATIVE:** Heel Lifts (p. 101) Turned-Out Squats (p. 108) **ALTERNATIVE:** Parallel Squats (p. 109) **STANDING CHAIR STRETCHES** Standing Chair Ankle Circles (p. 138) **ALTERNATIVE:** Heel Lifts (p. 139) Foot Towel Stretch (p. 120) **ALTERNATIVE:** Four Parts of the Foot (p. 121) Single-Leg Squats (p. 142) **ALTERNATIVE:** Squats (p. 143)

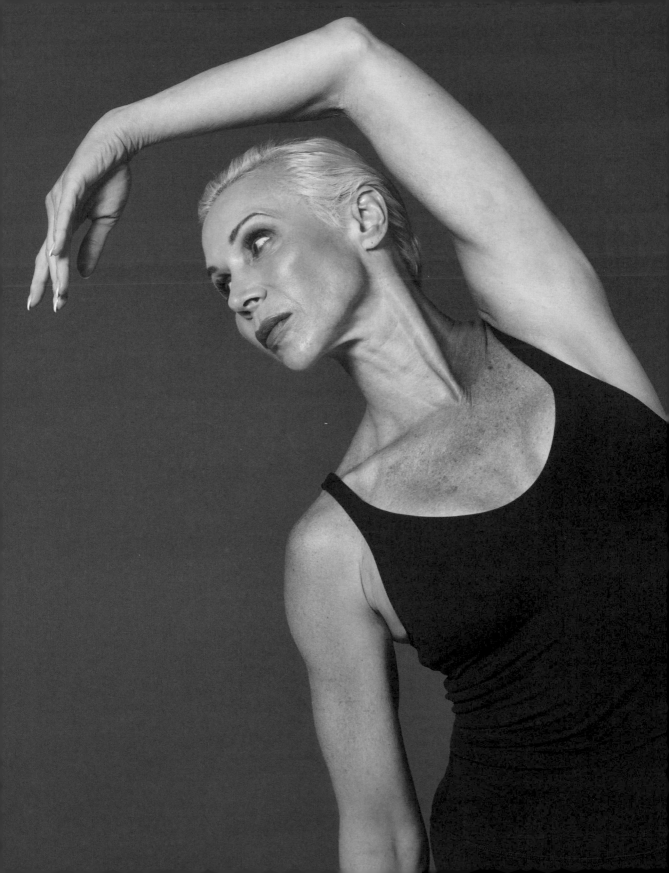

CHAPTER 03

The 28-Day Plans

Twenty-eight days is a great period during which to jump-start forming new daily habits, which is why this program is the perfect tool for changing your routine so you can keep pain at bay for good. Having trained many clients, I have seen that those who committed to this time frame were significantly more successful than those who did not. We learn best through repetition—repeating the same thing over and over makes the skill become easier. By the time you complete one of these plans, you won't have to think about every detail of every stretch. The movement will transition from your conscious thoughts, where you may need to revisit the movement instructions, to your subconscious. This will decrease the amount of time needed for each exercise. When you are able to do an exercise without having to review its cues, add a challenging exercise. But only add when you feel fully prepared to do so!

HOW TO PICK YOUR PLAN

Pain isn't a one-size-fits-all problem, which is why you will see a total of four 28-day plans for you to individualize for your needs. Each plan was built to help you create a routine that fits with your schedule and your unique area of pain. Whether you select the full-body plan or one of the pain-specific options, you can be confident that you'll get the pain relief you need. The plans are as follows:

FULL-BODY PLAN (p. 44)

PAIN-SPECIFIC PLANS:
NECK AND SHOULDER PLAN (p. 52)
LOWER BACK, HIPS, LEGS, AND FEET PLAN (p. 56)
SHOULDERS, ARMS, AND HANDS PLAN (p. 61)

The most effective plan is one you can actually stick to, so select your plan based on the time you can commit. As little as five minutes a day can do wonders for your aches. You'll reap even greater benefits by dedicating more time, so if you can do 15 minutes daily, go for it!

If you have just 5 minutes per day:
Select one of the pain-specific plans based on the area of pain you're experiencing.

If you have 10 minutes per day:
Select the full-body plan.

If you have 15 minutes per day:
Select the full-body plan plus one of the pain-specific plans based on the area of pain you're experiencing.

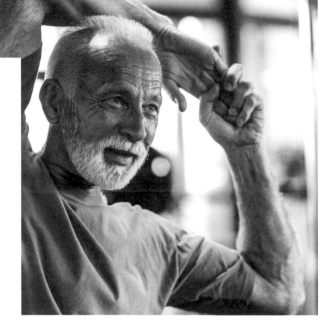

No matter which plan you choose, you'll spend one week on bed stretches, one on post-shower stretches, one on seated chair stretches, and one on the stretches you find most beneficial for your pain. As you progress from week to week and move stretches from the bed to right after the shower and then to the chair, you may continue with the post-shower exercises if you enjoy them, in addition to that week's prescribed stretches. Remember: This program is yours to make your own. Find what works for you. Begin with a plan that suits you. If you are distracted by pain or tightness in a specific area, begin there! Remember this is YOURS.

Use the base stretches if you begin to find the alternative stretches easy. You may add them to your list after the original exercise or replace the alternative stretch with the base stretches. You'll notice each stretch comes with a "Try It" recommendation. These simple suggestions will help you find little ways to use the exercises during your daily routine so you can sneak in a soothing stretch even when you don't think you have the time.

Working out even five minutes a day may be exhausting. Rest is as important to maximum health as working out. While 10 minutes a day seems like it wouldn't fatigue you, it can and will. Respect your natural cues. If you're tired, rest.

If you feel fantastic and are moving through the stretches easily, add another exercise to the routine. If you need more stretching in one body area or it feels good, go ahead and give that area a little more love. But only repeat the exercise one or two more times. Too much of a good thing is still too much.

Once you complete the 28-day plan you have chosen, my wish for you is that you will have incorporated these stretches into your daily activities and want to continue using this book to make your life better every day! Continue to do the stretches that feel great for you and look for stretching opportunities in your daily routine. I love integrating a simple stretch wherever I am. Going up and down the stairs? Stretch your Achilles tendon with a few heel lower-and-lifts at the step's edge. Putting groceries on a high shelf offers an opportunity for a few side-to-side stretches when done safely! The possibilities are endless. Finding stretches on your own brings awareness and focus and changes your movement, promoting better health and less daytime stiffness.

Must-Do Exercises for the Feet, Ankles, Wrists, and Hands

Everyone should focus on hand, wrist, ankle, and foot exercises, which affect our ability to accomplish many daily tasks and functions. You can do a few of these every day, no matter where you are in the program—think of them as bonus stretches. These include:

BED STRETCHES
Ankle Stretch (p. 79)
Flex, Extend, and Circle (p. 77)

POST-SHOWER STRETCHES
Heel Lifts (p. 139)
Parallel Squats (p. 109)

SEATED CHAIR STRETCHES
Four Parts of the Foot (p. 121)
Full-Body Stretch with Arm Arcs (p. 114)
Foot Towel Stretch (p. 120)

STANDING CHAIR STRETCHES
Heel Lifts (p. 139)
Four Parts of the Foot (p. 141)
Squats (p. 143)

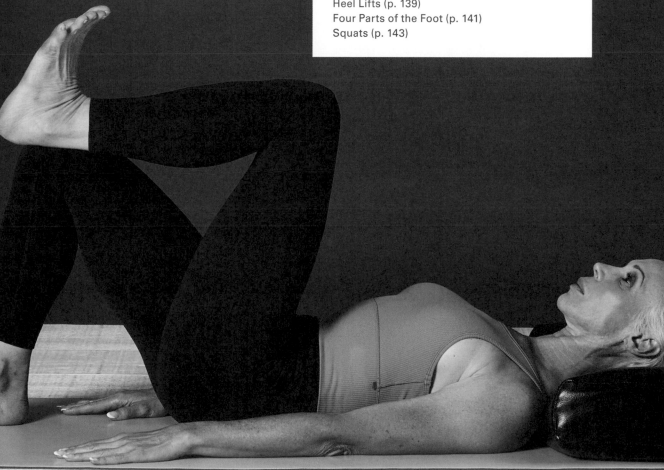

▶ FULL-BODY PLAN
DAYS 1-7

BED STRETCHES

Do the stretches in order, switching to the Alternative Stretches as needed. Additionally, pick **one** "Try It" stretch per day.

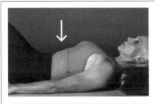

Progressive Breathing (p. 70)

Alternative Stretch:
Deep Breathing (p. 71)

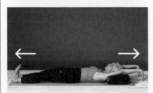

Full-Body Stretch with Arm Arcs (p. 74)

Alternative Stretch:
The Two-Way Stretch (p. 75)

TRY IT
Stretch your arms overhead while putting groceries away

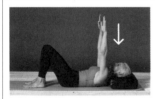

Shoulder Drops (p. 76)

Alternative Stretch:
Flex, Extend, and Circle (p. 77)

TRY IT
Move your shoulders back and forth while pushing a door open

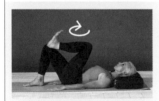

Lying Ankle Circles (p. 78)

Alternative Stretch:
Ankle Stretch (p. 79)

TRY IT
Circle your ankles while sitting at your kitchen table

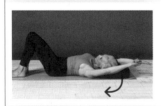

Side Stretch Legs Bent (p. 80)

Alternative Stretch:
Side-to-Side Stretch (p. 81)

TRY IT
Stretch to the side while reach for a high shelf

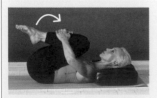

Double-Knee Hug (p. 82)

Alternative Stretch:
Single-Knee Hug (p. 83)

TRY IT
Hug your knees while putting on socks

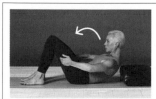

Roll-Up Back Stretch (p. 84)

Alternative Stretch:
Knee Circle Hug (p. 85)

TRY IT
Roll up as you sit up to get out of bed

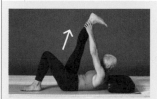

Climb a Tree (p. 86)

Alternative Stretch:
Hamstring Stretch (p. 87)

TRY IT
Stretch your leg while putting body lotion on

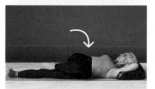

Single-Leg Twists (p. 88)

Alternative Stretch:
Windshield Wipers (p. 89)

TRY IT
Twist your body while getting in or out of a car

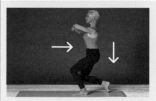

Single-Leg Back Squat (p. 90)

Alternative Stretch:
Standing Squat (p. 91)

TRY IT
Squat while pushing a grocery cart

FEEL-GOOD ADD-ONS

If you'd like a little more, try one (or all) of these soothing stretches.

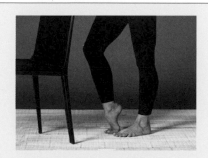

Running in Place Heels Down (p. 140)

Alternative Stretch:
Four Parts of the Foot (p. 141)

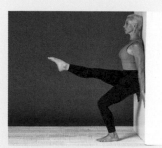

Single-Leg Squats (p. 142)

Alternative Stretch:
Squats (p. 143)

FULL-BODY PLAN
DAYS 8-14

POST-SHOWER STRETCHES

Do the stretches in order, switching to the Alternative Stretches as needed.
Additionally, pick **one** "Try It" stretch per day.

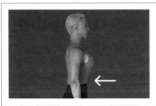

Progressive Breathing (p. 70)

Alternative Stretch:
Deep Breathing (p. 71)

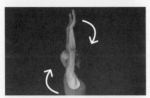

Full-Body Stretch with Arm Arcs (p. 94)

Alternative Stretch:
Two-Way Stretch (p. 95)

`TRY IT`
Washing the shower walls

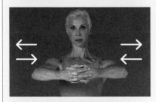

Shoulder Rolls (p. 96)

Alternative Stretch:
Alternating Arm Arcs (p. 97)

`TRY IT`
When brushing your hair, one shoulder at a time

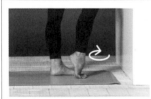

Finger Pull-Push (p. 98)

Alternative Stretch:
Flex and Fist (p. 99)

`TRY IT`
Putting on gloves

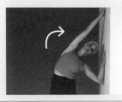

Standing Ankle Circles (p. 100)

Alternative Stretch:
Heel Lifts (p. 101)

`TRY IT`
Going up stairs

Side Bend (p. 102)

Alternative Stretch:
Side Stretch (p. 103)

`TRY IT`
Putting dishes away on a high shelf

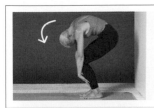

The Roll Down (p. 104)

Alternative Stretch:
Standing Upper Back Stretch (p. 105)

TRY IT
Washing
your legs

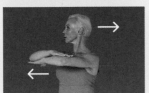

Genie Twist (p. 106)

Alternative Stretch:
Twist with One Hand on the Wall (p. 107)

TRY IT
While cooking
or vacuuming

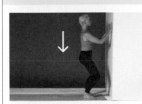

Turned-Out Squats (p. 108)

Alternative Stretch:
Parallel Squats (p. 109)

TRY IT
Sitting onto
a chair

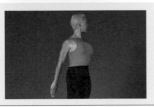

Chest Expansion with Head Turn (p. 110)

Alternative Stretch:
Chest Expansion without Head Turn (p. 111)

TRY IT
Crossing the
street and
looking both
ways

FEEL-GOOD ADD-ONS

If you'd like a little more, try one (or all) of these soothing stretches.

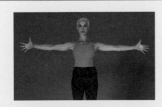

Spread Eagle (p. 146)

Alternative Stretch:
**Passive Shoulder
Stretches** (p. 147)

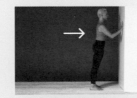

**Wall Pushups with
Elbows by Ribs** (p. 148)

Alternative Stretch:
**Wall Pushups with Elbows
Out** (p. 149)

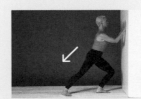

One-Leg Back Lunge
(p. 150)

Alternative Stretch: **One-Leg
Back Squat** (p. 151)

FULL-BODY PLAN
DAYS 15-21

SEATED CHAIR STRETCHES

Do the stretches in order, switching to the Alternative Stretches as needed. Additionally, pick **one** "Try It" stretch per day.

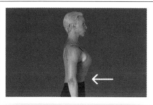

Progressive Breathing (p. 70)

Alternative Stretch:
Deep Breathing (p. 71)

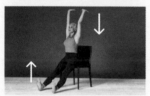

Full-Body Stretch with Arm Arcs (p. 114)

Alternative Stretch:
Two-Way Stretch (p. 115)

TRY IT
As an hourly break while working

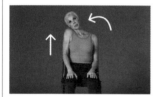

Ear and Shoulder Taps (p. 116)

Alternative Stretch:
Yes and No (p. 117)

TRY IT
Before crossing the street

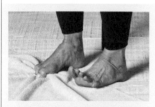

Foot Towel Stretch (p. 120)

Alternative Stretch:
Four Parts of the Foot (p. 121)

TRY IT
Walking up or down stairs

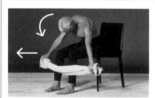

Forward Stretch Seated with Towel with Twist (p. 124)

Alternative Stretch:
Forward Stretch Seated with Towel (p. 125)

TRY IT
After showering

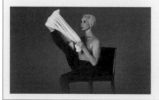

Hamstring Stretch with Towel (p. 126)

Alternative Stretch:
Single-Knee Lifts with Towel (p. 127)

TRY IT
Washing your legs

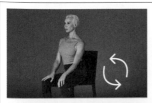

Bottoms Up, Down, and Around (p. 128)

Alternative Stretch:
Bottoms Up and Down (p. 129)

`TRY IT`
**Sitting
watching TV**

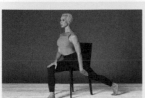

Thigh and Hip Stretch (p. 130)

Alternative Stretch:
Thigh and Hip Stretch with Bent Legs (p. 131)

`TRY IT`
**Sitting while
working**

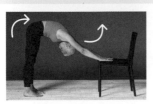

Extended Cat (p. 134)

Alternative Stretch:
Cat and Cow (p. 135)

`TRY IT`
**Making
the bed**

FEEL-GOOD ADD-ONS

If you'd like a little more, try one (or all) of these soothing stretches.

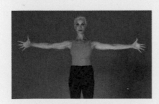

Spread Eagle (p. 146)

Alternative Stretch:
**Passive Shoulder
Stretches** (p. 147)

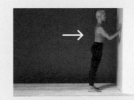

**Wall Pushups with
Elbows by Ribs** (p. 148)

Alternative Stretch:
**Wall Pushups with Elbows
Out** (p. 149)

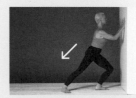

One-Leg Back Lunge
(p. 150)

Alternative Stretch: **One-Leg
Back Squat** (p. 151)

FULL-BODY PLAN
DAYS 22-28

YOUR CHOICE

Do your favorite series of stretches from the last three weeks and record them in the first column below. Additionally, pick **one** "Try It" stretch from that same series each day and record it in the second column.

	TRY IT
	TRY IT
	TRY IT
	TRY IT
	TRY IT
	TRY IT
	TRY IT
	TRY IT
	TRY IT
	TRY IT

FEEL-GOOD ADD-ONS

If you'd like a little more, try one (or all) of these soothing stretches.

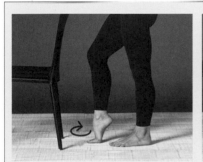

Standing Chair Ankle Circles (p. 138)

Alternative Stretch: **Heel Lifts** (p. 139)

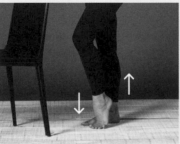

Running in Place Heels Down (p. 140)

Alternative Stretch: **Four Parts of the Foot** (p. 141)

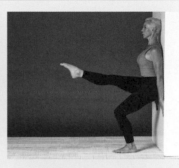

Single-Leg Squats (p. 142)

Alternative Stretch: **Squats** (p. 143)

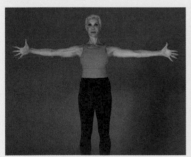

Spread Eagle (p. 146)

Alternative Stretch: **Passive Shoulder Stretches** (p. 147)

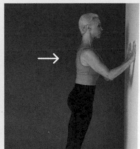

Wall Pushups with Elbows by Ribs (p. 148)

Alternative Stretch: **Wall Pushups with Elbows Out** (p. 149)

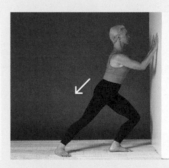

One-Leg Back Lunge (p. 150)

Alternative Stretch: **One-Leg Back Squat** (p. 151)

▶ NECK AND SHOULDER PLAN
DAYS 1-7

BED STRETCHES

Do the stretches in order, switching to the Alternative Stretches as needed.
Additionally, pick **one** "Try It" stretch per day.

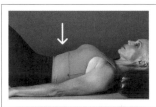

Progressive Breathing (p. 70)

Alternative Stretch:
Deep Breathing (p. 71)

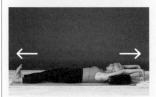

Full-Body Stretch with Arm Arcs (p. 74)

Alternative Stretch:
The Two-Way Stretch (p. 75)

TRY IT
Stretch your arms overhead while putting groceries away

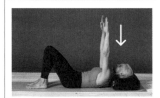

Shoulder Drops (p. 76)

Alternative Stretch:
Flex, Extend, and Circle (p. 77)

TRY IT
Move your shoulders back and forth while pushing a door open

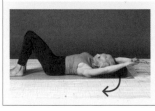

Side Stretch Legs Bent (p. 80)

Alternative Stretch:
Side-to-Side Stretch (p. 81)

TRY IT
Stretch to the side while reach for a high shelf

Note
If moving your neck is painful, omit the neck-specific exercises. The other exercises will stretch and strengthen your neck as well as your shoulders.

DAYS 8-14

POST-SHOWER STRETCHES

Do the stretches in order, switching to the Alternative Stretches as needed.
Additionally, pick **one** "Try It" stretch per day.

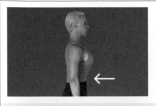

Progressive Breathing (p. 70)

Alternative Stretch:
Deep Breathing (p. 71)

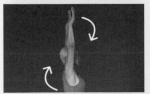

Full-Body Stretch with Arm Arcs (p. 94)

Alternative Stretch:
Two-Way Stretch (p. 95)

TRY IT
Washing the
shower walls

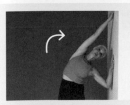

Shoulder Rolls (p. 96)

Alternative Stretch:
Alternating Arm Arcs (p. 97)

TRY IT
When brushing
your hair,
one shoulder
at a time

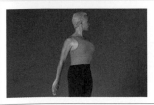

Side Bend (p. 102)

Alternative Stretch:
Side Stretch (p. 103)

TRY IT
When putting
something on
a high shelf

Chest Expansion with Head Turn (p. 110)

Alternative Stretch:
Chest Expansion without Head Turn (p. 111)

TRY IT
When crossing
a street and
looking both
ways

NECK AND SHOULDER PLAN
DAYS 15-21

SEATED CHAIR STRETCHES

Do the stretches in order, switching to the Alternative Stretches as needed. Additionally, pick **one** "Try It" stretch per day.

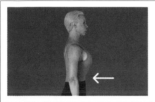

Progressive Breathing (p. 70)

Alternative Stretch:
Deep Breathing (p. 71)

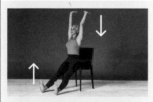

Full-Body Stretch with Arm Arcs (p. 114)

Alternative Stretch:
Two-Way Stretch (p. 115)

TRY IT
As an hourly break

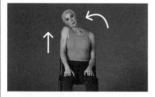

Ear and Shoulder Taps (p. 116)

Alternative Stretch:
Yes and No (p. 117)

TRY IT
When watching TV

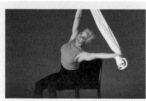

Seated Side-to-Side Stretch with Towel (p. 122)

Alternative Stretch:
Seated Simple Side-to-Side Stretch with Towel (p. 123)

TRY IT
Stretch to the side and twist while fixing your review mirror

DAYS 22-28

YOUR CHOICE

Do your favorite series of stretches from the last three weeks and record them in the first column below. Additionally, pick **one** "Try It" stretch from that same series each day and record it in the second column.

	TRY IT
	TRY IT
	TRY IT
	TRY IT
	TRY IT
	TRY IT
	TRY IT
	TRY IT
	TRY IT
	TRY IT

►LOWER BACK, HIPS, LEGS, AND FEET PLAN
DAYS 1-7

BED STRETCHES

Do the stretches in order, switching to the Alternative Stretches as needed. Additionally, pick **one** "Try It" stretch per day.

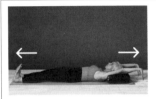

Full-Body Stretch with Arm Arcs (p. 74)

Alternative Stretch:
The Two-Way Stretch (p. 75)

TRY IT
Putting groceries away

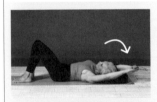

Side Stretch Legs Bent (p. 80)

Alternative Stretch:
Side-to-Side Stretch (p. 81)

TRY IT
Reaching for a high shelf

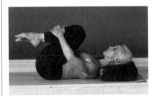

Double-Knee Hug (p. 82)

Alternative Stretch:
Single-Knee Hug (p. 83)

TRY IT
Putting on socks

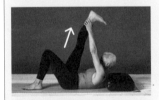

Climb a Tree (p. 86)

Alternative Stretch:
Hamstring Stretch (p. 87)

TRY IT
When putting lotion on your legs

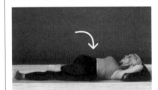

Single-Leg Twists (p. 88)

Alternative Stretch:
Windshield Wipers (p. 89)

TRY IT
Getting in and out of a car

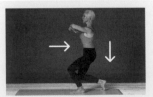

Single-Leg Back Squat (p. 90)

Alternative Stretch:
Standing Squat (p. 91)

TRY IT
Pushing a grocery cart

DAYS 8-14

POST-SHOWER STRETCHES

Do the stretches in order, switching to the Alternative Stretches
as needed. Additionally, pick **one** "Try It" stretch per day.

	Full-Body Stretch with Arm Arcs (p. 94) Alternative Stretch: **Two-Way Stretch** (p. 95)	**TRY IT** **Washing the shower walls**
	Side Bend (p. 102) Alternative Stretch: **Side Stretch** (p. 103)	**TRY IT** **When putting items away on a high shelf**
	The Roll Down (p. 104) Alternative Stretch: **Standing Upper Back Stretch** (p. 105)	**TRY IT** **When drying your legs**
	Genie Twist (p. 106) Alternative Stretch: **Twist with One Hand on the Wall** (p. 107)	**TRY IT** **Vacuuming**
	Turned-Out Squats (p. 108) Alternative Stretch: **Parallel Squats** (p. 109)	**TRY IT** **Sitting onto a chair**

LOWER BACK, HIPS, LEGS, AND FEET PLAN
DAYS 15-21

SEATED CHAIR STRETCHES

Do the stretches in order, switching to the Alternative Stretches as needed. Additionally, pick **one** "Try It" stretch per day.

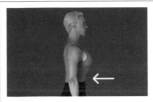

Progressive Breathing (p. 70)

Alternative Stretch:
Deep Breathing (p. 71)

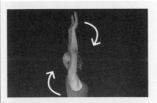

Full-Body Stretch with Arm Arcs (p. 114)

Alternative Stretch:
Two-Way Stretch (p. 115)

TRY IT
As an hourly break

Ear and Shoulder Taps (p. 116)

Alternative Stretch:
Yes and No (p. 117)

TRY IT
When working on the computer or watching TV

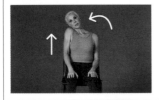

Foot Towel Stretch (p. 120)

Alternative Stretch:
Four Parts of the Foot (p. 121)

TRY IT
After showering, while standing on a bath mat

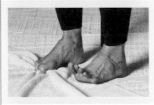

Seated Side-to-Side Stretch with Towel (p. 122)

Alternative Stretch:
Seated Simple Side-to-Side Stretch with Towel (p. 123)

TRY IT
Fixing your rearview mirror

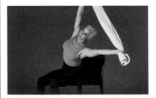

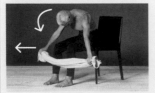

Forward Stretch Seated with Towel with Twist (p. 124)

Alternative Stretch:
Forward Stretch Seated with Towel (p. 125)

TRY IT
Stretch to the side and twist while fixing your review mirror

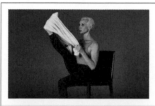

Hamstring Stretch with Towel (p. 126)

Alternative Stretch:
Single-Knee Lifts with Towel (p. 127)

`TRY IT`
**Sitting on
the couch with
a blanket**

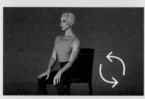

Bottoms Up, Down, and Around (p. 128)

Alternative Stretch:
Bottoms Up and Down (p. 129)

`TRY IT`
**Sitting
watching TV**

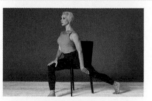

Thigh and Hip Stretch (p. 130)

Alternative Stretch:
Thigh and Hip Stretch with Bent Legs (p. 131)

`TRY IT`
**Pushing a
door open**

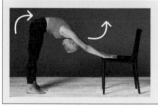

Extended Cat (p. 134)

Alternative Stretch:
Cat and Cow (p. 135)

`TRY IT`
Making the bed

LOWER BACK, HIPS, LEGS, AND FEET PLAN
DAYS 22-28

YOUR CHOICE

Do your favorite series of stretches from the last three weeks and record them in the first column below. Additionally, pick **one** "Try It" stretch from that same series each day and record it in the second column.

	TRY IT
	TRY IT
	TRY IT
	TRY IT
	TRY IT
	TRY IT
	TRY IT
	TRY IT
	TRY IT
	TRY IT

SHOULDERS, ARMS, AND HANDS PLAN
DAYS 1-7

BED STRETCHES

Do the stretches in order, switching to the Alternative Stretches
as needed. Additionally, pick **one** "Try It" stretch per day.

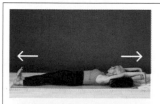

Full-Body Stretch with Arm Arcs (p. 74)

Alternative Stretch:
The Two-Way Stretch (p. 75)

TRY IT
Stretch your
arms while
taking a shirt
off overhead

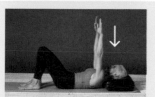

Shoulder Drops (p. 76)

Alternative Stretch:
Flex, Extend, and Circle (p. 77)

TRY IT
Move your
shoulders back
and forth
while pushing
a door open

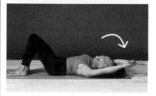

Side Stretch Legs Bent (p. 80)

Alternative Stretch:
Side-to-Side Stretch (p. 81)

TRY IT
Stretch to the
side while reach
for a high shelf

SHOULDERS, ARMS, AND HANDS PLAN
DAYS 8-14

POST-SHOWER STRETCHES

Do the stretches in order, switching to the Alternative Stretches as needed. Additionally, pick **one** "Try It" stretch per day.

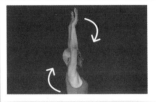

Full-Body Stretch with Arm Arcs (p. 94)

Alternative Stretch:
Two-Way Stretch (p. 95)

TRY IT
Washing the shower walls

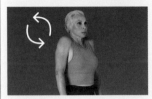

Shoulder Rolls (p. 96)

Alternative Stretch:
Alternating Arm Arcs (p. 97)

TRY IT
As an hourly break

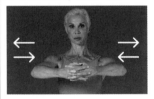

Finger Pull-Push (p. 98)

Alternative Stretch:
Flex and Fist (p. 99)

TRY IT
When washing hands

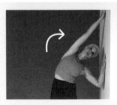

Side Bend (p. 102)

Alternative Stretch:
Side Stretch (p. 103)

TRY IT
When putting on a sweater

DAYS 15-21

SEATED CHAIR STRETCHES

Do the stretches in order, switching to the Alternative Stretches as needed. Additionally, pick **one** "Try It" stretch per day.

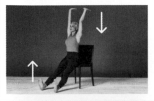

Full-Body Stretch with Arm Arcs (p. 114)

Alternative Stretch:
Two-Way Stretch (p. 115)

TRY IT
As an hourly break

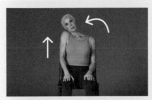

Ear and Shoulder Taps (p. 116)

Alternative Stretch:
Yes and No (p. 117)

TRY IT
When on the computer or watching TV

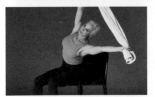

Seated Side-to-Side Stretch with Towel (p. 122)

Alternative Stretch:
Seated Simple Side-to-Side Stretch with Towel (p. 123)

TRY IT
With a scarf when getting ready to go out

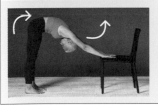

Extended Cat (p. 134)

Alternative Stretch:
Cat and Cow (p. 135)

TRY IT
Making the bed

SHOULDERS, ARMS, AND HANDS PLAN
DAYS 22-28

YOUR CHOICE

Do your favorite series of stretches from the last three weeks and record them in the first column below. Additionally, pick **one** "Try It" stretch from that same series each day and record it in the second column.

	TRY IT
	TRY IT
	TRY IT
	TRY IT
	TRY IT
	TRY IT
	TRY IT
	TRY IT
	TRY IT
	TRY IT

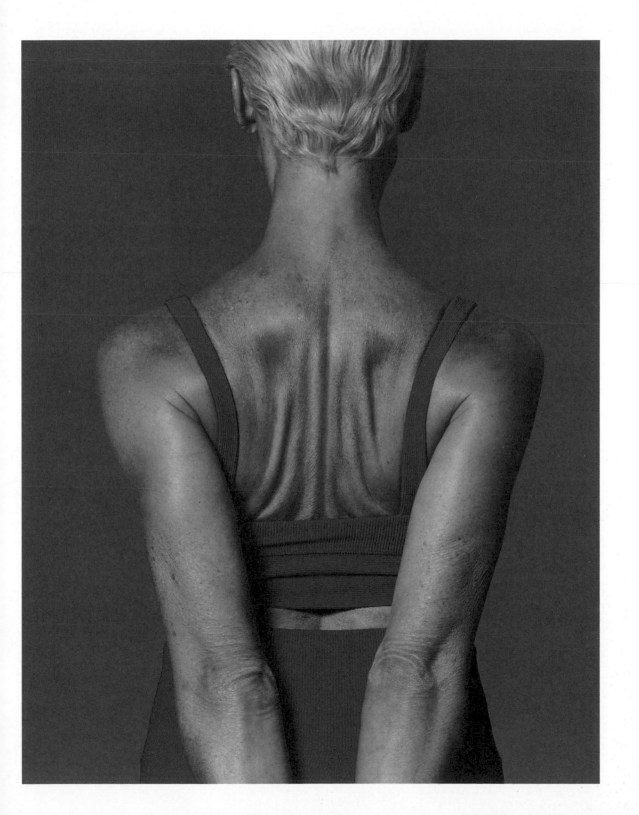

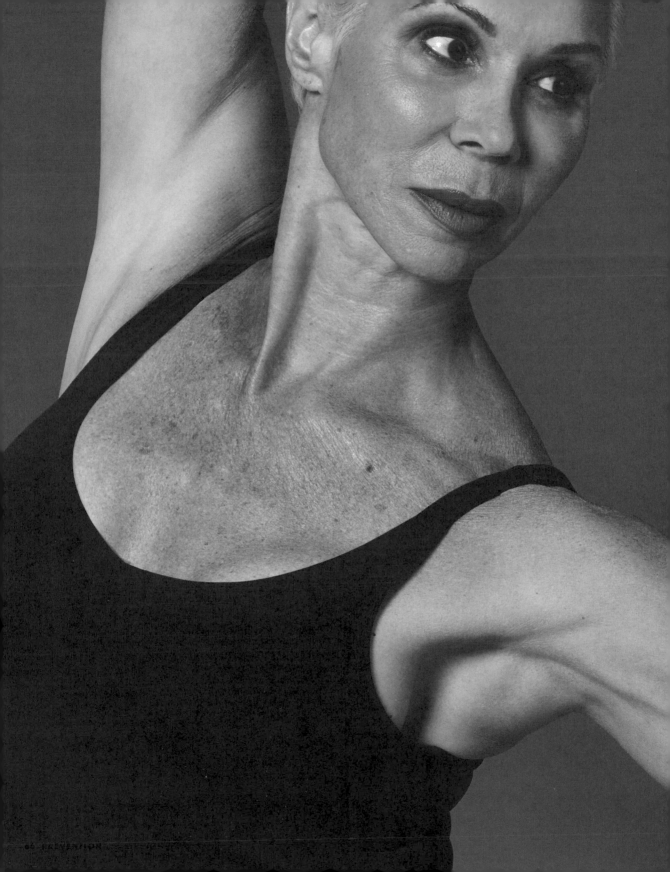

CHAPTER 04

Stretching Glossary

Here you'll find 75 stretches organized by when you should do them: in bed, sitting, standing, or after showering. As mentioned earlier, you will see many exercises by the same name throughout multiple categories—they are the same stretch but done in different places and positions. This repetition will help your brain hardwire the stretches so they become second nature. Plus, performing a stretch in multiple places helps you learn the stretch and all its nuances, and helps you move more easily in everyday life as you adapt the moves in new and valuable ways. Review the key body positions listed in the box on the next page, then read each of the exercises that are new to you three times before you begin.

WHAT YOU'LL NEED

You don't need much to complete the stretching routines in this program, but make sure you have access to the following:

BED

SHOWER

HIGH-BACKED CHAIR

WALL

STANDARD-SIZE BATH TOWEL
(it can be from 20 x 40 inches to 28 x 54 inches, so not a hand towel)

Key Body Positions

If you're reading a stretch and wondering, "What the heck does this mean?" use this list to find the answer. Take a few minutes to review the terms below, as many refer to ways to stand during the stretches.

EVERSION OF THE FOOT: When the foot's bottom or sole faces away from the midline, or the vertical center of your body (imagine a line running through the center of your body from head to toe).

INVERSION OF THE FOOT: When the foot's bottom or sole faces the body's midline, or the vertical center of your body.

PARALLEL LEGS: Stand or sit with your legs apart, keeping your knees in line with the center of your hips and your heels. Your toes point forward and your knees align with the second toe.

SHOULDER HEIGHT: When you lift one or both arms, the arm(s) will be parallel to the ground.

SIT BONES OR SITTING BONES: Also known as your ischial tuberosities, these two bony points are located in the lower middle part of the buttocks and are what hurt when you sit on a hard chair.

SIT-BONE-WIDTH APART: Stand with your heels and the center of the ball of your foot in line with your sit bones.

STOMACH IN AND UP (DIAPHRAGM): Without allowing the ribs to pop forward, pull your navel back toward your spine and feel your stomach muscles lift to support your back. Remember to breathe!

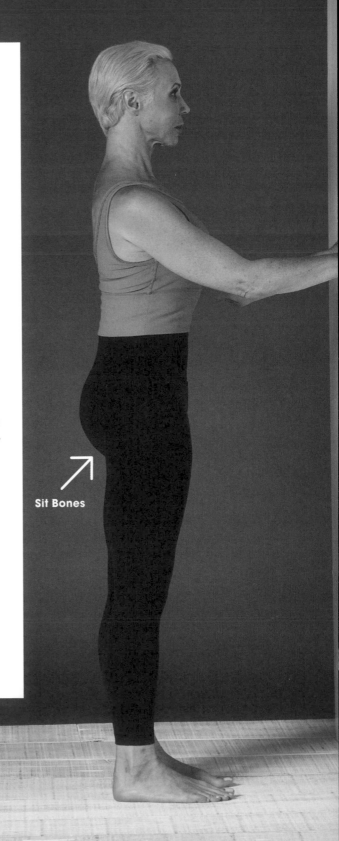

Sit Bones

ELEMENTS OF EACH EXERCISE

For each exercise series, you'll see this outline:

TRY THIS FOR

This section indicates what bodily pain the exercise helps alleviate, although it may help elsewhere too.

WHERE YOU SHOULD FEEL IT

Here you'll learn where you should feel the stretch in your body. If you feel a burning or pinching pain in these places or elsewhere, then stop. Listen to this signal.

STARTING POSITION

This is your foundation for entering and ending each stretch from a place of stability. It may also include additional instruction for your starting position if it varies from the usual basic starting position.

POSTURAL CHECK-IN

Many exercises also include what I call a Postural Check-in. Because we so often fall out of alignment without being aware of it, I've added these little reminders to realign your body so you get the most from the exercise. You might find yourself shifting your body to avoid stretching precisely the body part that needs to be stretched, so keep an eye out for the patterns you fall into.

In general, always line up your joints as well as you can when moving, while you stretch and in everyday life. Then, use the Postural Check-Ins to clarify how you're lying, sitting, and standing. Use the photos to assist you in understanding what proper alignment looks like.

Breathwork

Every stretching series in this book begins the same way: with a few deep breaths. This will not only send a signal to your body to relax, but will also serve as a familiar point from which to start your daily routine. No matter how you're stretching—lying down, after showering, standing, or seated—begin with one of these soothing breathwork exercises.

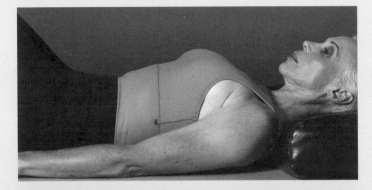

PROGRESSIVE BREATHING

TRY IT FOR
General tension

WHERE YOU SHOULD FEEL IT
Rib cage

STARTING POSITION
Lying down, seated, or standing

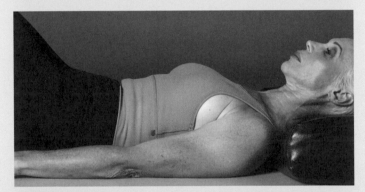

1 Inhale deeply for five counts. Try to fill your lungs and not breathe with your belly, expanding your rib cage as you inhale.

2 Exhale fully for five counts, emptying your lungs and not breathing with your belly. Pull your stomach in as if you are zipping up those tight jeans. Depress your rib cage as you exhale, visualizing a towel around your ribs being pulled tighter and squeezing the air out.

3 Inhale deeply for six counts—try to fill your lungs, expand your rib cage, and not breathe with your belly. Zip your jeans!

4 Exhale fully for six counts, emptying your lungs. Your rib cage is depressed as you exhale.

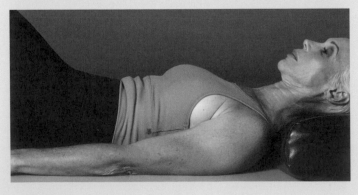

5 Repeat deep inhalation and full exhalation, adding one count with each repetition. Build to a 12-count breath over the course of the plan, adding a count every other day. Execute the relevant Postural Check-In for the stretch series. See post-shower (p. 93), seated (p. 113), standing at a chair (p. 137), or standing at the wall (p. 145).

➡➡ TOO CHALLENGING?
See opposite page for an easier option.

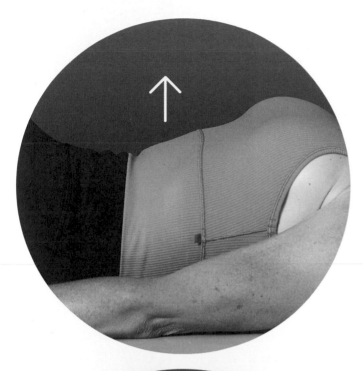

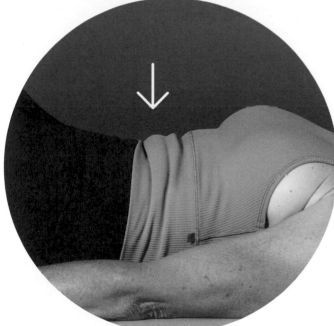

ALTERNATIVE STRETCH
DEEP BREATHING

TRY IT FOR
General tension

WHERE YOU SHOULD FEEL IT
Rib cage

STARTING POSITION
Lying down, seated, or standing

1 Inhale through your nose deeply for five counts. Fill your lungs. Your rib cage should expand to the sides like an accordion. Your navel pulls in and up, and your spine is long. Pause with your lungs full for two counts.

2 Exhale for six counts through softly parted lips. Exhale more air than you took in. Squeeze the air out like wringing out a washcloth. Pause with your lungs empty for two counts.

3 Repeat three times slowly. Execute the relevant Postural Check-In for the stretch series. See post-shower (p. 93), seated (p. 113), standing at a chair (p. 137), or standing at the wall (p. 145).

Tip
You may fill a balloon on the exhalation or blow a pinwheel to help you fully empty the lungs.

Bed Stretches

Warm up before you rise! You should wake up your brain and body before you begin your day. This series will help you do just that, and it will prepare you for easy and comfortable movement morning to night. You'll begin with some gentle deep breathing then gradually work your way to standing. Think about this as the breakfast for your day's movement!

These morning stretches are the foundation for all the exercises in this book. If your bed is too small for you to lie with your legs straight and arms overhead, lie diagonally across it. Use a pillow or two where and when it is suggested. Most of the stretches in this section begin in the same rest position (right) or some variation of it. We won't worry about Postural Check-Ins for most of this series, as all but one of these stretches are done lying down.

➡➡ BED BREATHWORK

Always start the bed stretches series with either of the breathwork exercises from pages 70 and 71.

REST POSITION

This is a comfortable position with your knees bent and head supported.

1 Lie on your back with your head on a pillow that supports your head and neck. Don't let the pillow lift your head too much. Your head should be high enough that your neck is long and continues the spine's curve, yet your throat remains open.

2 Bend your knees so they point to the ceiling and are sit-bone-width apart; your feet should be flat on the bed, toes pointing forward. Put a pillow under your knees for support if that feels more comfortable.

3 Extend your arms along your sides with soft elbows. Place palms down.

4 Gently inhale and exhale 10 slow breaths.

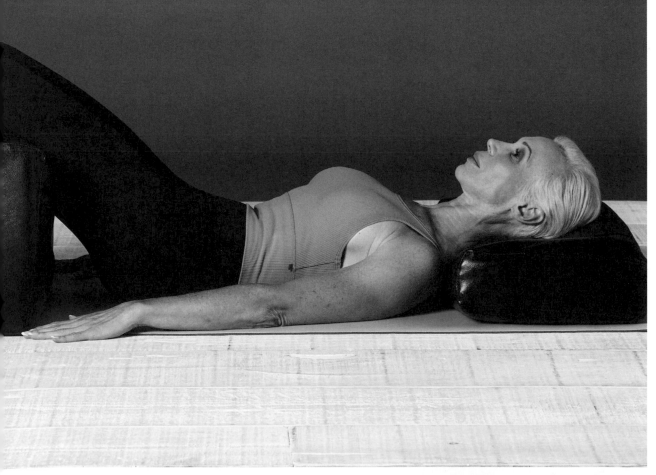

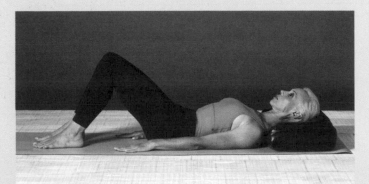

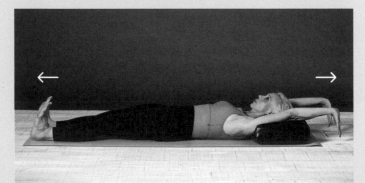

FULL-BODY STETCH WITH ARM ARCS

TRY IT FOR
Stiffness through the entire body

WHERE YOU SHOULD FEEL IT
Entire body

STARTING POSITION
Rest Position
Lie in the middle of your bed with a pillow under your head only. If your bed is too short for you to extend both arms and legs simultaneously, stretch your arms first and then stretch your legs.

1 On a deep inhalation through your nose, reach your arms overhead, toward the top of the bed. Stretch your legs straight toward the bottom of the bed. Spread your fingers and toes as wide as possible.

2 Pull your toes toward your knees and press your palms away from your head, with fingers pointing to the bed.

3 Stretch in two directions. Push through your heels and flex your feet and hands. Don't arch your lower back. Hold the stretch for three counts.

4 Exhale and stop flexing your hands and feet. Pull your stomach toward your spine to protect your lower back. Bend your knees, lift your arms to the ceiling, then place your arms at your sides.

5 Repeat these moves twice, then return to the Rest Position.

➡ TOO CHALLENGING?
See opposite page for an easier option.

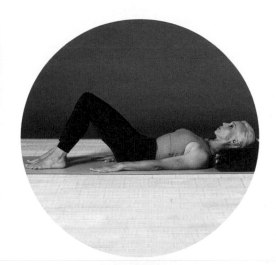

ALTERNATIVE STRETCH
THE TWO-WAY STRETCH

TRY IT FOR
Stiffness through the entire body

WHERE YOU SHOULD FEEL IT
Entire body

STARTING POSITION
Rest Position
Lie in the middle of your bed with a pillow under your head only. If your bed is too short for you to extend both arms and legs simultaneously, stretch your arms first and then stretch your legs.

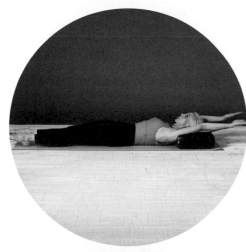

1 On a deep inhalation through your nose, reach your arms overhead, toward the top of the bed, and stretch your legs straight toward the bottom of the bed. Spread your fingers and toes as wide as possible.

2 Pull your toes toward your knees and press your palms away with your fingers pointing toward the bed.

3 Stretch in two directions, pushing through your heels and pressing your palms away, flexing your feet and hands. Hold the stretch for three counts.

4 Exhale through softly parted lips and relax, with arms overhead and legs straight.

5 Repeat the two-way stretch twice. Then bring your arms to your sides to finish and bend your knees to return to the Rest Position.

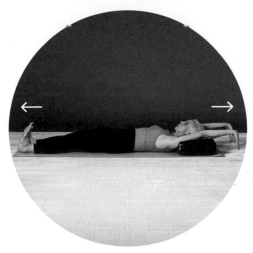

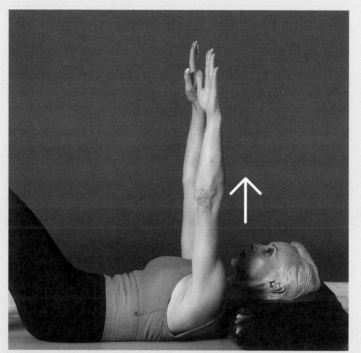

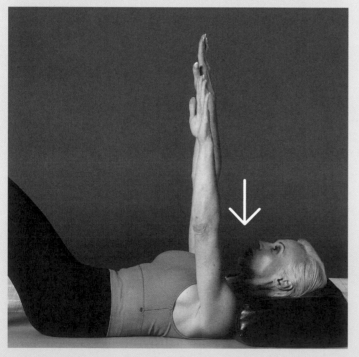

SHOULDER DROPS

TRY IT FOR
Neck and shoulders

WHERE YOU SHOULD FEEL IT
Neck, shoulders, and upper back

STARTING POSITION
Rest Position

1 Inhale and lift both arms up toward the ceiling.

2 Reach your right arm up as if you are trying to touch the ceiling, allowing both shoulders to peel off the bed.

3 Hold and deepen your reach for three counts.

4 Release the stretch and allow your right shoulder to "drop" back onto the bed.

5 Repeat the reaching movement with the left arm, alternating right and left for a total of three sets of drops.

6 Return to the Rest Position.

➤➤ TOO CHALLENGING?
See opposite page for an easier option.

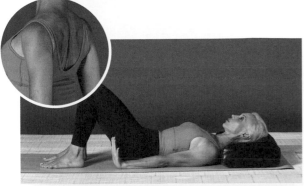

ALTERNATIVE STRETCH
FLEX, EXTEND, AND CIRCLE

TRY IT FOR
Neck, shoulders, wrists, and fingers

WHERE YOU SHOULD FEEL IT
Neck, shoulders, arms, wrists, and fingers

STARTING POSITION
Rest Position
With a pillow under your head and a pillow underneath your knees, if needed.

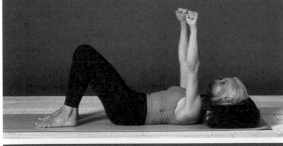

1 Inhale deeply.

2 Exhale and flex your hands. Keeping your arms on the bed by your sides, bend your wrists to lift your hands toward the ceiling, fingers spread. Press your palms toward the end of the bed. Arms remain extended by your sides and on the bed.

3 Hold the press for three counts.

4 Inhale and press your palms down onto the bed with spread fingers.

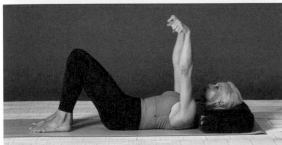

5 As palms press down, try to touch your shoulder blades together behind you and open your chest. (See inset photo.)

6 Repeat two times.

7 Inhale and lift your arms to shoulder height in front of you, toward the ceiling.

8 Inhale and clench your hands into tight fists.

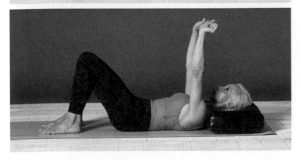

9 Circle your wrists three times slowly toward each other and three times away from each other.

10 Return to Rest Position.

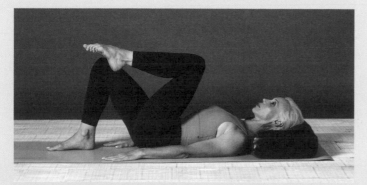

LYING ANKLE CIRCLES

TRY IT FOR
Ankles, feet, and toes

WHERE YOU SHOULD FEEL IT
Ankles, feet, and toes

STARTING POSITION
Rest Position

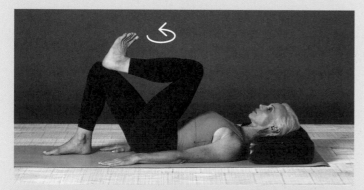

1 Bend one leg toward your chest to lift the foot, folding the knee to the chest a little closer than a 90-degree angle. Keep your knee, hip, and foot in line with each other.

2 Circle the ankle of the lifted foot in three slow circles to the right, as if tracing the edge of the circle with your pinkie toe. Move only the foot and ankle. Then do three slow circles to the left.

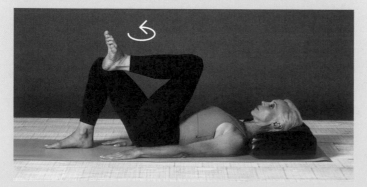

3 Place your foot down and repeat on the other side. Return to Rest Position.

➡ **TOO CHALLENGING?**
See opposite page for an easier option.

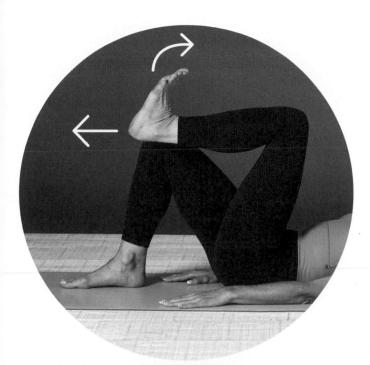

ALTERNATIVE STRETCH
ANKLE STRETCH

TRY IT FOR
Ankles, feet, and toes

WHERE YOU SHOULD FEEL IT
Ankles, feet, and toes

STARTING POSITION
Rest Position

1 Bend your right knee toward your chest to lift your foot, with the knee slightly closer than a 90-degree angle. Keep your knee, hip, and foot in line with each other.

2 Flex the right foot and push your heel away, then point and stretch the top of your foot. Relax. Repeat the flex-and-point two times before ending with your foot flexed.

3 Lift the inner edge of your right foot, so the bottom of the foot moves toward your left leg. Then lift the outer edge of the foot so that the bottom of your foot moves away from your left leg.

4 Repeat, alternating the inversion to eversion three times. Return to Rest Position, then repeat on the left leg.

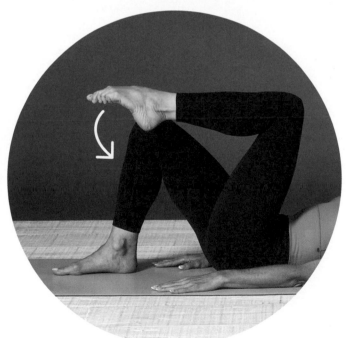

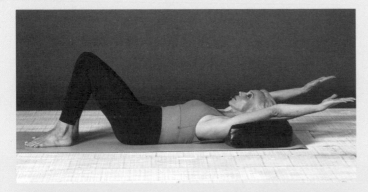

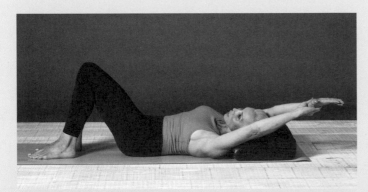

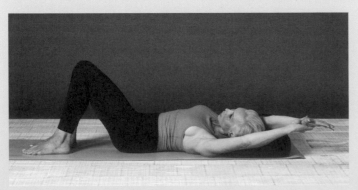

SIDE STRETCH LEGS BENT

TRY IT FOR

Shoulders, waist, hands, and wrists

WHERE YOU SHOULD FEEL IT

Waist, hands, shoulders, and entire side body

STARTING POSITION

Rest Position

Lie in the center of your bed. If your bed is too short for you to extend both arms and legs simultaneously, stretch your arms first and then stretch your legs.

1 Reach your arms up to the ceiling and then toward the top of the bed, the backs of your hands facing the bed, and fingers spread with palms toward the ceiling. Pull your stomach in toward your spine as you increase the stretch of both arms toward the top of the bed.

2 Inhale and stretch the right side of your body, reaching further overhead with the right hand. Use your left hand to grasp the right wrist below the wrist joint. Pull the right wrist to increase the right-side stretch. Your upper body will be in a left-curved banana shape. Hold for three counts.

3 Release the pull and center your body. Change hands and grasp the left wrist with the right hand and pull with the right hand to stretch the left side for three counts.

4 Relax and let go of any tension. Repeat two times, alternating stretches side to side. Return to Rest Position.

➡ TOO CHALLENGING?

See opposite page for an easier option.

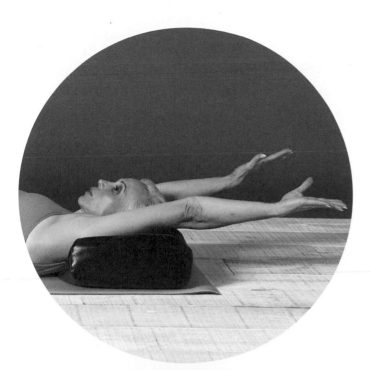

ALTERNATIVE STRETCH
SIDE-TO-SIDE STRETCH

TRY IT FOR
Shoulders, waist, lower back, hands, and wrists

WHERE YOU SHOULD FEEL IT
Waist, hands, shoulders, and entire side of body

STARTING POSITION
Rest Position

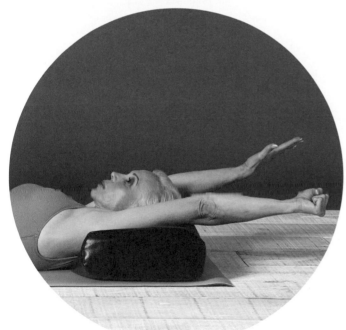

1 Reach your arms up to the ceiling and then toward the top of the bed, the backs of your hands facing the bed, and fingers spread with palms toward the ceiling. Pull your stomach in toward your spine as you increase the stretch of both arms toward the top of the bed.

2 Inhale and reach overhead with your right hand as if stretching for an apple on a high tree branch. Exhale and grasp the apple by making a fist with your right hand. Press the fist even further away from you.

3 Inhale and spread the fingers of your right hand and relax the reach. Exhale and let both arms relax.

4 Repeat on the left side, then repeat twice, alternating sides. Return to Rest Position.

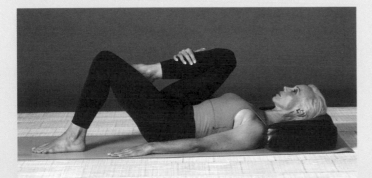

DOUBLE-KNEE HUG

TRY IT FOR
Lower back and hips

WHERE YOU SHOULD FEEL IT
Back of the legs, lower back, and hips

STARTING POSITION
Rest Position

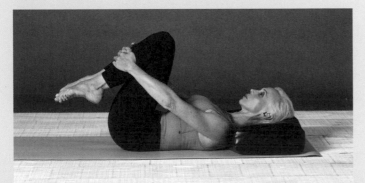

1 Bend your right knee toward your chest, lifting your foot and folding your leg into your chest, and place your right hand on your shin. (If you have bad knees, hold each leg under the thigh.) Then bend your left knee toward your chest to position your left foot next to your right foot, and place your left hand on the left shin.

2 Hug your thighs toward and against your chest by pulling on your shins with your hands. Open your elbows to the sides, then release your hands to allow your thighs to move off your torso.

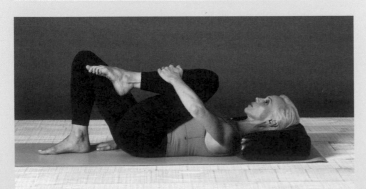

3 Repeat the hug-and-release two times. After the last release, take your right hand off your right shin to place your right foot down, followed by the left. Return to Rest Position.

➼ TOO CHALLENGING?
See opposite page for an easier option.

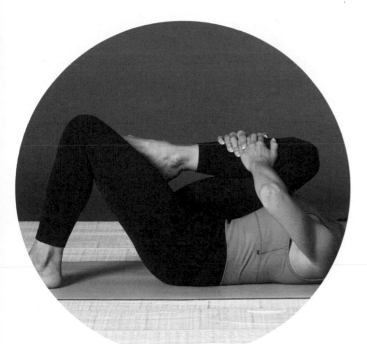

ALTERNATIVE STRETCH
SINGLE-KNEE HUG

TRY IT FOR
Lower back and hips

WHERE YOU SHOULD FEEL IT
Back of the legs, lower back, and hips

STARTING POSITION
Rest Position

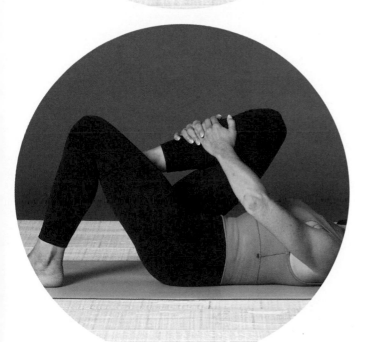

1 Bend your right knee toward your chest to lift your foot, folding your thigh to your chest. Place both hands on your shin. (If you have bad knees, hold each leg under the thigh.) Hug the thigh toward your chest and against your torso by pulling it with your hands, with your elbows open to the sides. Hold the hug for three counts.

2 Release your hands and allow your thigh to move off your torso.

3 Pull your hands against your shin again, hugging your thigh toward your chest for three counts. Release your hands and allow your thigh to move off your torso.

4 Release your hands and place your arms along the sides of your body. Return the right foot onto the bed into the Rest Position.

5 Repeat on the left side. Return to Rest Position.

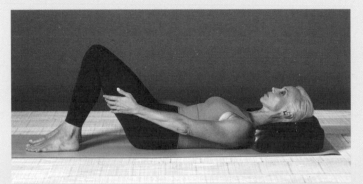

ROLL-UP BACK STRETCH

TRY IT FOR
Lower back and hips

WHERE YOU SHOULD FEEL IT
Back of the legs, lower back, hips, and abdominals

STARTING POSITION
Rest Position

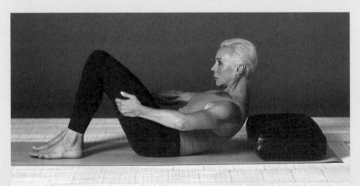

1 Inhale and place your hands on the back of your thighs with elbows open to the sides. Hold your thighs with your hands. Lift your head off the pillow by pulling with your arms, and direct your gaze to your stomach.

2 Exhale, pull with your hands against your thighs to lift your shoulders and curl your upper body up and off the bed. Bend your elbows as you roll up. If there's tension in your neck, place one hand behind your head and support your head to relax your neck.

3 Hold this position for three counts, then reverse the action to lie back down.

4 When your head is down, move your hands from your thighs and place them along the side of your body. Rest three counts.

5 Repeat three times. If you're using a hand to support the weight of your head, alternate which hand holds your head each repetition. Return to Rest Position.

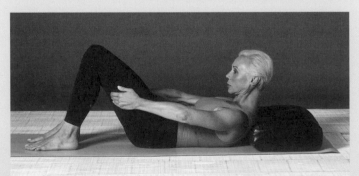

➡ TOO CHALLENGING?
See opposite page for an easier option.

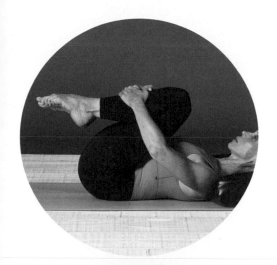

ALTERNATIVE STRETCH
KNEE CIRCLE HUG

TRY IT FOR
Lower back and hips

WHERE YOU SHOULD FEEL IT
Back of the legs, lower back, and hips

STARTING POSITION
Rest Position

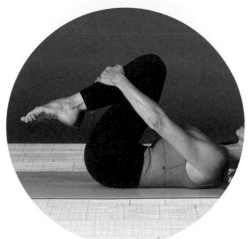

1 Bend your right knee toward your chest, lifting your foot and folding your leg into your chest. Place your right hand on your shin. (If you have bad knees, hold each leg under the thigh.)

2 Bend your left knee toward your chest, lifting your foot and folding your leg into your chest. Place your left hand on your shin. Hug both legs to your chest.

3 Make three small circles to the right with both legs, keeping your hands on your shins.

4 Pause with knees centered, hug your knees deeper into your chest, and make three small circles to the left. Pause with knees centered and hug both knees deeper into your chest.

5 Release the hug. Place your right foot, then your left foot down. Return to Rest Position.

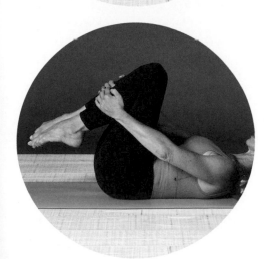

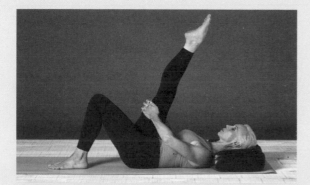

CLIMB A TREE

TRY IT FOR
Lower back and hips

WHERE YOU SHOULD FEEL IT
Back of the legs

STARTING POSITION
Rest Position

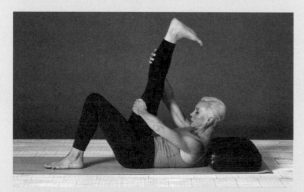

1 Place both hands on the back of your right thigh, pulling your thigh to your chest. Point your foot softly, and move your knee so it points to the space between your shoulder and your ear. Open and lift your elbows to each side as you pull. Hold your leg to your chest for three counts.

2 Without moving your thigh, gently extend your leg toward the ceiling as much as possible, maintaining the soft point of your foot. Flex your foot, bringing your toes toward your knee and pushing your heel out.

3 Use your arms to lift your head and your shoulders off the bed, bending your elbows as needed and curling your upper body up. There should be no tension in your neck.

4 Keeping your hips and shoulders parallel, walk your hands up your leg as high as possible without straining and without allowing your sides to twist. Hold for three counts.

5 Push your heel away to increase the stretch, then point your foot, reaching your toes away from your knee. Repeat the flex and toe point twice with the right foot.

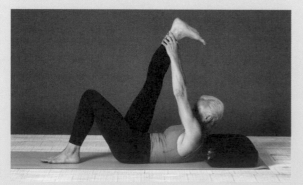

6 Walk your hands down the "tree" and resume holding your thigh. Lower your shoulders and head, then bend your knee and place your foot down.

7 Return to the Rest Position. Repeat stretch on the other side, then return to Rest Position.

➦ TOO CHALLENGING?
See opposite page for an easier option.

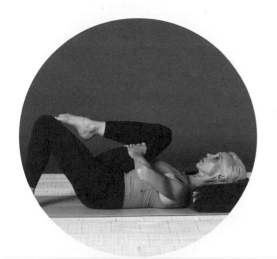

ALTERNATIVE STRETCH
HAMSTRING STRETCH

TRY IT FOR
Lower back and hips

WHERE YOU SHOULD FEEL IT
Back of your legs and glutes

STARTING POSITION
Rest Position

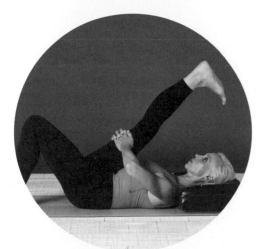

1 Bend your right knee toward your chest to lift your softly pointed foot. Your knee should point toward the space between your shoulder and your ear, with both hands holding the back of your thigh.

2 Pull your thigh to your chest, with elbows open and lifted to the side. Hold your leg to your chest for three counts.

3 Without moving your thigh, gently extend your leg toward the ceiling as much as possible, keeping your foot softly pointed. Flex your foot by bringing your toes toward your knee and pushing out with your heel. Then point your foot by reaching your toes away from your knee.

4 Repeat the flex and point of your right foot twice.

5 Place the foot down, release your hands, and return to the Rest Position.

6 Repeat on the other side, then return to the Rest Position.

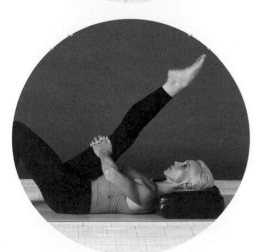

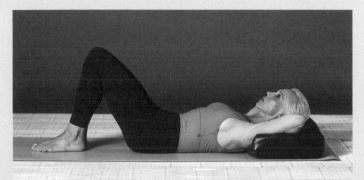

SINGLE-LEG TWISTS

TRY IT FOR
Lower back, upper back, shoulders, and neck

WHERE YOU SHOULD FEEL IT
Inner thighs, hips, front of hips, waist, and lower back

STARTING POSITION
Rest Position
Place a pillow between your thighs if needed.

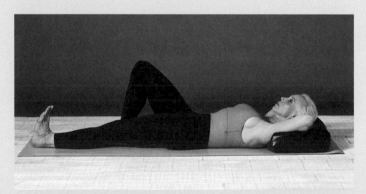

1 Clasp your hands behind your head and press your elbows open gently. Pull your navel toward your spine to keep your back straight.

2 Inhale and slide your left foot forward to straighten the leg. Flex your foot, pulling your toes toward your knee.

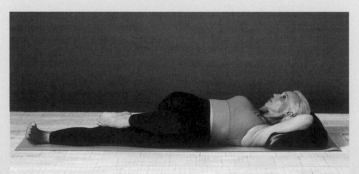

3 Exhale and twist your right knee across your left leg. Lift your right hip as you cross your right knee over your left leg. Hold for three counts. Pull your navel toward your spine and keep your back straight.

4 Point your right knee straight up. Bend your left leg to repeat on the other side. Alternate legs for two sets of twists then return to Rest Position.

➡️ TOO CHALLENGING?
See opposite page for an easier option.

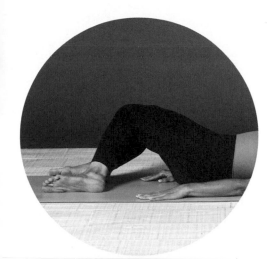

ALTERNATIVE STRETCH
WINDSHIELD WIPERS

TRY IT FOR
Lower back, hips, and inner thighs

WHERE YOU SHOULD FEEL IT
Inner thighs, hips, front of hips, waist, and lower back

STARTING POSITION
Rest Position

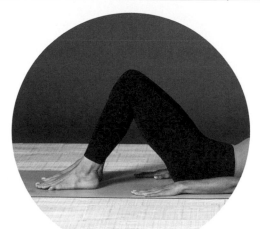

1 Place your arms by your sides, palms down. Your arms and shoulders should align from center finger to center finger.

2 Gently rock knees side to side, letting your feet move as needed; feel as if the wind is blowing your legs. Do not move from the shoulders up.

3 Repeat three to five times, side to side.

4 End in the Rest Position with feet and legs together.

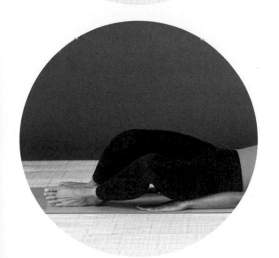

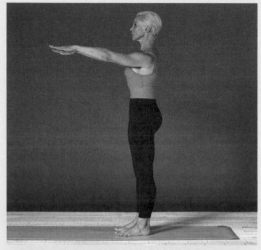

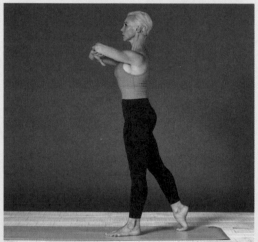

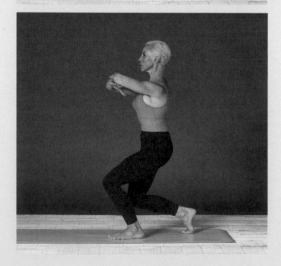

SINGLE-LEG BACK SQUAT

TRY IT FOR

Knees, ankles, lower back, and hips

WHERE YOU SHOULD FEEL IT

Thighs, glutes, calves, and front of hips

STARTING POSITION

Standing

By now you should feel ready to get out of bed. Begin this stretch standing with your legs sit-bone-width apart and parallel, heels under the hips and feet pointing forward. Let your arms hang by your sides, elbows soft.

1 Lift your arms to shoulder height in front of you, then fold your arms, fingertips to elbows. Keep your knees unlocked. Keeping both legs in line with your sit bones, move your right leg back with a lifted heel, in line with its sit bone and the center of the ball of its foot.

2 Shift your body weight to the front leg, keeping shoulders and hips parallel to each other. Inhale and bend both knees, pulling your stomach in to protect your spine. Bend your front knee over, but not past, your toes. Bend your back knee directly down. Exhale and extend your legs.

3 Repeat three times, then step the back leg forward and repeat on the left side. To finish, step the back leg forward so you're standing with your legs a little more than sit-bone-width apart. Lower your arms. Execute a Post-Shower Postural Check-In (page 93).

➡️ TOO CHALLENGING?
See opposite page for an easier option.

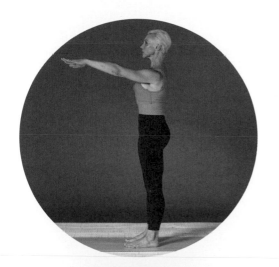

ALTERNATIVE STRETCH
STANDING SQUAT

TRY IT FOR

Knees, ankles, lower back, and hips

WHERE YOU SHOULD FEEL IT

Thighs, glutes, and calves

STARTING POSITION

Standing

Stand with your legs sit-bone-width apart and parallel, with heels under your hips and feet pointing forward, keeping your knees soft. Let your arms hang by your sides, elbows soft.

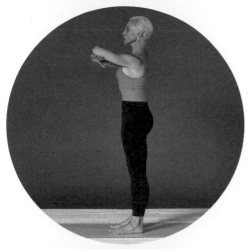

1 Lift your arms to shoulder height in front of you, palms facing the floor. Fold your arms, fingertips to elbows.

2 Inhale and bend your knees, pulling your stomach in. Your knees should extend over, but not past, your toes. Try to keep your heels down, although they may lift. Exhale and straighten your legs.

3 Repeat three times. Lower your arms to your sides to finish. Execute a Post-Shower Postural Check-In (page 93).

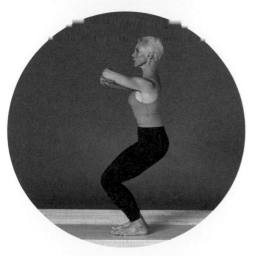

Post-Shower Stretches

Time to hit the shower! Stretching after a warm shower helps melt away pain, as warm water pre-heats your body, even your muscles. Your muscles are like gelatin, which contains collagen. Each muscle fiber in your body consists of 1% to 10% of this protein. Like chilled gelatin, cold muscle fibers are thick, dense, and solid. But when it's warm, gelatin is fluid and moves easily. In the shower, your muscles can become more flexible thanks to the warmth. (Don't make the water too hot, or you may become dizzy.)

Perform these stretches right after your shower on a non-slip surface while your muscles are still warm. Once you feel comfortable with these moves, feel free to try them in your shower with the warm water on. These work best in a walk-in shower where you can place your hands on the wall opposite the showerhead while still being in range of the running water. You should also have an easy-to-reach support to grab if you need it, and your shower floor should have a non-slip surface big enough for you to stand on with your feet about a foot apart.

Wherever you do them, be sure to constantly check your posture. For these stretches, the Postural Check-In is also the starting position (except where noted). So as you start, take an extra moment to ensure you're aligned. And I also ask you to end with a Postural Check-In after each exercise. We're trying to bring your focus to your alignment.

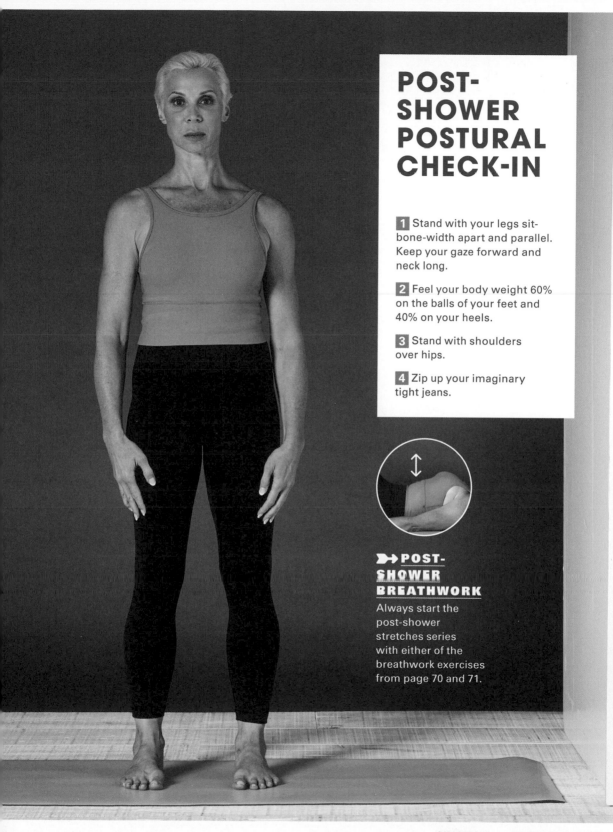

POST-SHOWER POSTURAL CHECK-IN

1 Stand with your legs sit-bone-width apart and parallel. Keep your gaze forward and neck long.

2 Feel your body weight 60% on the balls of your feet and 40% on your heels.

3 Stand with shoulders over hips.

4 Zip up your imaginary tight jeans.

➤ POST-SHOWER BREATHWORK

Always start the post-shower stretches series with either of the breathwork exercises from page 70 and 71.

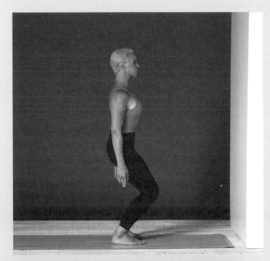

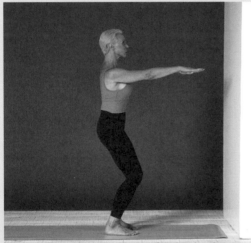

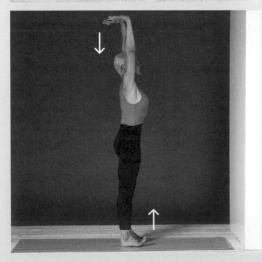

FULL-BODY STRETCH WITH ARM ARCS

TRY IT FOR
Stiffness throughout the entire body

WHERE YOU SHOULD FEEL IT
Entire body

STARTING POSITION
Standing
Stand with legs sit-bone-width apart and parallel, toes pointing forward. Zip up your imaginary tight jeans to pull your stomach in and protect your spine. Your heels, glutes, upper back, and, if possible, the back of your head, should touch the wall.

1 Bend your knees softly over your second toes. On a deep inhalation, lift your arms forward to shoulder height and then overhead.

2 While the arms arc, straighten your legs and spread your fingers and toes. Stretch in two directions, pushing through your heels and pressing your palms toward the ceiling. Hold the stretch for three counts.

3 Exhale and stop flexing your hands. Bend your knees and lower your arms along your side body. Return to the Starting Position.

4 Repeat twice, then execute a Post-Shower Postural Check-In (page 93).

➡ TOO CHALLENGING?
See opposite page for an easier option.

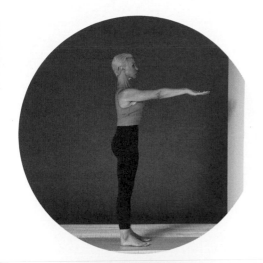

ALTERNATIVE STRETCH
TWO-WAY STRETCH

TRY IT FOR
Stiffness throughout the entire body

WHERE YOU SHOULD FEEL IT
Entire body

STARTING POSITION
Standing
Stand with legs sit-bone-width apart and parallel, toes pointing forward. Zip up your imaginary tight jeans to pull your stomach in and protect your spine.

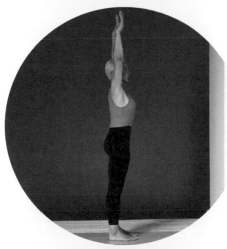

1 On a deep inhalation, lift your arms to shoulder height and then overhead toward the ceiling.

2 Spread your fingers and toes, then flex your feet and hands. Lift your toes and press your palms toward the ceiling. Stretch in two directions, pushing through your heels and pressing your palms up. Hold the stretch for three counts.

3 Exhale and stop flexing your hands and feet. Relax everything! Lower your arms to the sides of your body. Return to the Starting Position.

4 Repeat twice. Execute a Post-Shower Postural Check-In (page 93).

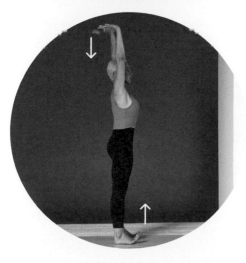

SHOULDER ROLLS

TRY IT FOR

Shoulders, upper back, and neck

WHERE YOU SHOULD FEEL IT

Shoulders and upper back

STARTING POSITION

Standing

➤➤ TOO CHALLENGING?

See opposite page for an easier option.

1 Inhale and lift your shoulders toward your ears. Pull your stomach in to protect your back, which should be straight. Circle your shoulders back and try to touch your shoulder blades together while opening your chest. Imagine you're wearing a tight vest to prevent your ribs from flaring.

2 Drop your shoulders down and as far away from your ears as possible, as if you're holding a heavy suitcase in each hand. Stretch your neck.

3 Roll your shoulders forward and allow your chest to close. Stretch your upper back, then reverse the movement to open your chest. That's one roll. Repeat two times, then reverse the movement to roll your shoulders three times in the opposite direction. Execute a Post-Shower Postural Check-In (page 93).

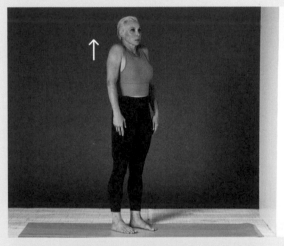

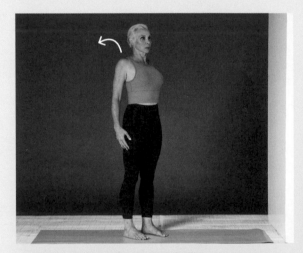

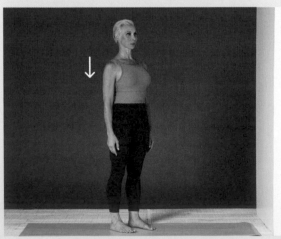

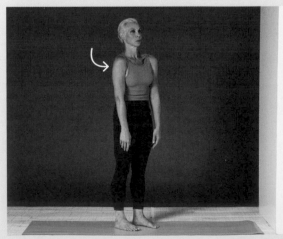

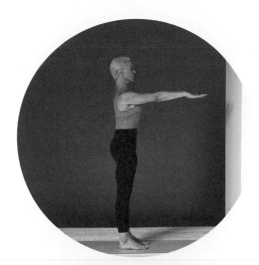

ALTERNATIVE STRETCH
ALTERNATING ARM ARCS

TRY IT FOR
Shoulders and neck

WHERE YOU SHOULD FEEL IT
Shoulders, upper back, ribs, and neck

STARTING POSITION
Standing
Stand with legs sit-bone-width apart and parallel, arms by your sides.

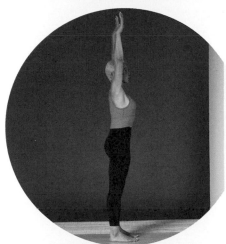

1 On a deep inhalation, lift your arms to shoulder height and then overhead toward the ceiling, fingers spread.

2 Lower the right arm and stretch the left arm up.

3 Exhale and switch arms. Repeat the switch five times. Bring both arms to shoulder height, then lower your arms to your sides. Execute a Post-Shower Postural Check-In (page 93).

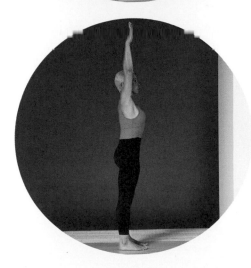

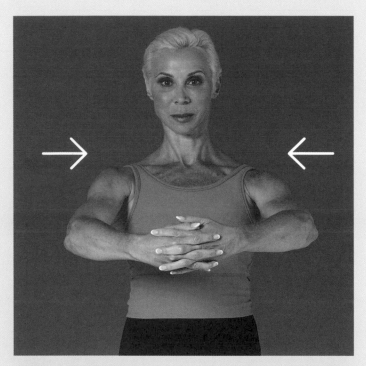

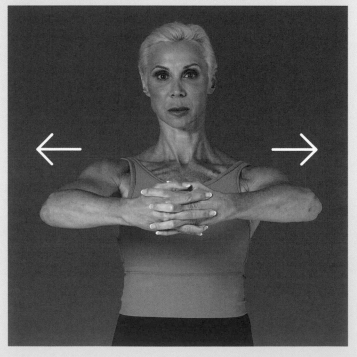

FINGER PULL-PUSH

TRY IT FOR
Wrists and hands

WHERE YOU SHOULD FEEL IT
Fingers, hands, wrists, upper arms, and chest

STARTING POSITION
Standing

If doing this stretch in the shower, execute with warm water running over your hands as you face the showerhead.

1 Interlace your fingers using your dominant grip (the way that feels most natural), with your palms facing you, at chest height. Bend your elbows to create a circle with your arms, as if hugging a tree.

2 Press your fingers together for three counts. Your fingers should grasp your hands and hold on for dear life.

3 Release the pressure on your hands, but not the grip, and pause. Without allowing the fingers to separate, try to pull your hands apart. Then grasp your fingers and hold on tight, again, for three to five counts. Release the pressure and pause.

4 Repeat the stretches twice, then repeat steps 1 to 4 with your non-dominant grip. Execute a Post-Shower Postural Check-In (page 93).

➡➡ TOO CHALLENGING?
See opposite page for an easier option.

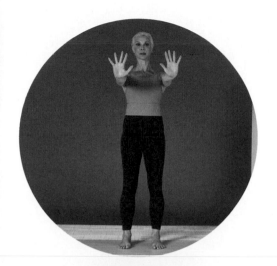

ALTERNATIVE STRETCH
FLEX AND FIST

TRY IT FOR
Wrists and hands

WHERE YOU SHOULD FEEL IT
Wrists and hands

STARTING POSITION
Standing

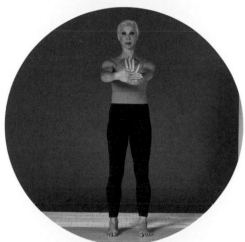

1 On a deep inhalation, lift both of your arms to shoulder height, in line with your shoulders, palms down. Flex your hands back and press your palms forward. Spread your fingers and hold for three counts.

2 Squeeze your hands into tight fists and hold for three counts. Repeat the spread fingers to fist motions three times. End with hands flexed, fingers long and together.

3 Lower your right hand to chest height, then shift it to the center so it lines up with middle of your chest.

4 Place your left fingers on the palm side of the right fingers, with your hands palm to palm. Your right fingers should point to the ceiling, and the left fingers should point to the right, so your hands create a cross. Gently press with the left hand to stretch the right palm back.

5 Release the pressure. Slide the left hand up, so the left palm is on the right fingers. Gently press with the left hand to stretch the right fingers back. Release the pressure. Take the left hand off the right hand.

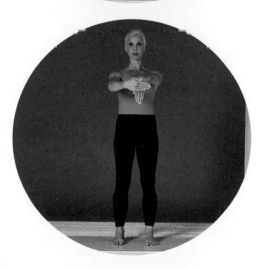

6 Point the right fingers down. Place your left palm onto the back of your right hand. Gently press with the left hand to stretch the right hand toward you. Release the pressure. Slide the left hand down, so the left palm is on the right fingers. Gently press with the left hand to stretch the right fingers toward you, then release the pressure.

7 Repeat the stretches twice, then repeat with the other hand. Execute a Post-Shower Postural Check-In (page 93).

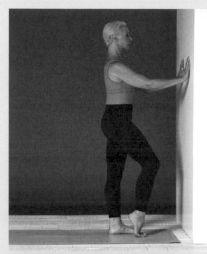

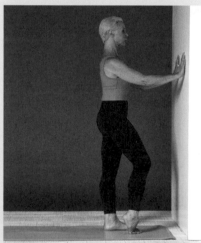

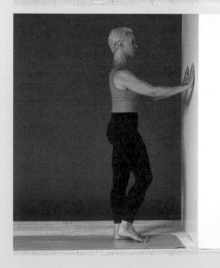

STANDING ANKLE CIRCLES

TRY IT FOR
Ankles and feet

WHERE YOU SHOULD FEEL IT
Ankles and feet

STARTING POSITION
Standing
Place your hands on the wall in front of you, fingertips at shoulder height with fingers pointed up and palms flat. Bend your elbows and point them down. Place your legs sit-bone-width apart and parallel, with knees facing forward toward the wall.

1 Bend your right knee and place the foot forward, on the ball of the foot with a lifted heel. Your foot should align with your knee, and your knee should align with your hip. Don't shift your hips or sink to one side; your shoulders and hips should form parallel lines.

2 Allow the heel to lower and lift as you circle the heel three times to the right and three times to the left.

3 Return to the starting position. Repeat with your other leg. Execute a Post-Shower Postural Check-In (page 93).

➡️ TOO CHALLENGING?
See opposite page for an easier option.

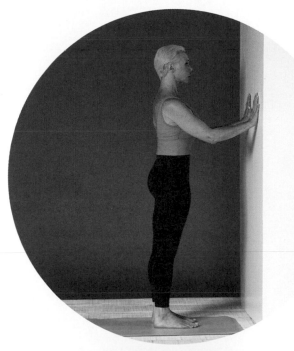

ALTERNATIVE STRETCH
HEEL LIFTS

TRY IT FOR
Ankles and feet

WHERE YOU SHOULD FEEL IT
Ankles, feet, thighs, and glutes

STARTING POSITION
Standing

Place your hands on the wall in front of you, fingertips at shoulder height with palms flat and fingers pointing up. Bend your elbows and point them down. Zip up those tight jeans. Position your legs so they are sit-bone-width apart and parallel, with knees and feet facing the wall.

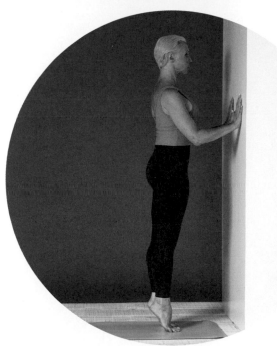

1 Lift your heels straight up as if a hand is pressing them up. Don't shift your heels out or in.

2 Hold the lift for three counts. Don't lock your knees or arch your back.

3 Slowly lower your heels with control. Repeat three times, then execute a Post-Shower Postural Check-In (page 93).

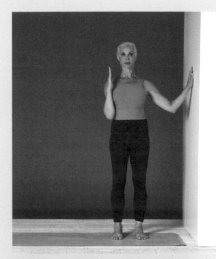

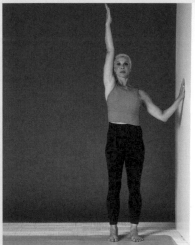

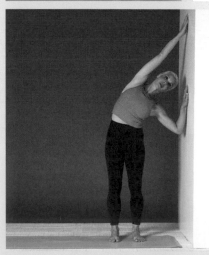

SIDE BEND

TRY IT FOR
Shoulders, waist, rib cage, lower back, upper back, and fingers

WHERE YOU SHOULD FEEL IT
Arms, shoulders, side body, and waist

STARTING POSITION
Standing

Stand sideways about one foot from the wall, with your left hand on the wall at shoulder height, and your elbow bent and down. Position your left hand slightly in front of your shoulder. Put your right arm down by your side. Stand with legs sit-bone-width apart and parallel, toes pointing forward.

1 Bend your right arm to bring your thumb in front of your right armpit, palm facing the wall. Extend the right arm straight up, pulling the stomach in, and reach the right arm toward the wall.

2 Stretch the side of your body to the right. Hold for three counts. Return to standing upright. Repeat the process one or two more times, then lower the right arm by bending the right arm to bring the thumb in front of your armpit, palm facing the wall.

3 Repeat on the left side, turning to place your right hand on the wall. Execute a Post-Shower Postural Check-In (page 93).

➥ TOO CHALLENGING?
See opposite page for an easier option.

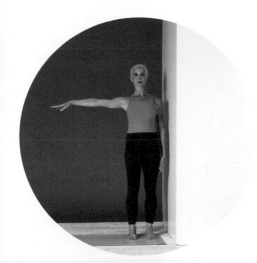

ALTERNATIVE STRETCH
SIDE STRETCH

TRY IT FOR

Shoulders, waist, rib cage, lower back, upper back, and fingers

WHERE YOU SHOULD FEEL IT

Arms, shoulders, side body, and waist

STARTING POSITION

Standing

Stand perpendicular to the wall with your left shoulder on the wall, arms by your sides. Place your legs sit-bone-width apart and parallel, toes pointing forward. Zip up your imaginary tight jeans to pull your stomach in and protect your spine.

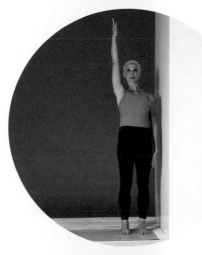

1 Lift your right arm to the side to shoulder height, but slightly in front of your shoulder, palm facing down.

2 Rotate your right arm so your palm faces the ceiling. Lift your right arm up to the side so your fingers point to the ceiling. Extend your right arm straight up, without locking the elbow, your palm facing the wall. Pull your stomach in and reach your right arm toward the wall until you can place the hand on the wall, if possible.

3 Slide the right hand up the wall. Keep your fingertips on the wall even if your palm comes off. Hold for three counts.

4 Reverse the action and slide your right hand down the wall to release the stretch. Then raise your right arm to the side, palm up. Rotate your arm so your palm faces down.

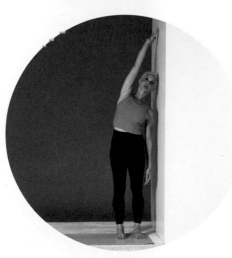

5 Lower your arm to return to the start position. Repeat twice.

6 Repeat on the left side, and return to the Starting Position. Execute a Post-Shower Postural Check-In (page 93).

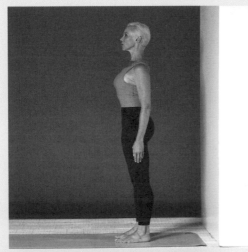

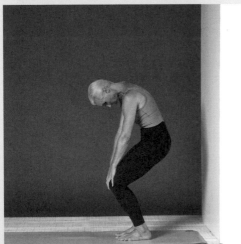

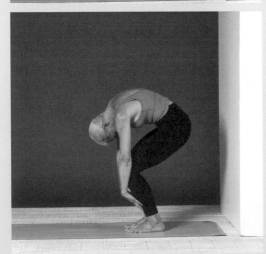

THE ROLL DOWN

TRY IT FOR
Lower back, upper back, and neck

WHERE YOU SHOULD FEEL IT
Lower back, upper back, neck, and abdominals

STARTING POSITION
Standing

1 Bend your knees softly and place your hands on your thighs. Pull your stomach in. Inhale and lower your head to bring your gaze to your hands.

2 Exhale and gradually roll your spine down, hands sliding down your legs as the upper and lower back stretch. Pause to pull your stomach in.

3 Reverse the action and roll up. Repeat twice. Execute a Post-Shower Postural Check-In (page 93).

➡ TOO CHALLENGING?
See opposite page for an easier option.

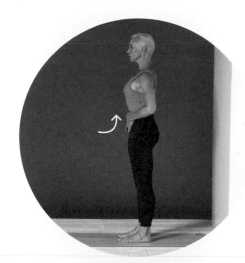

ALTERNATIVE STRETCH
STANDING UPPER BACK STRETCH

TRY IT FOR
Lower back, upper back, and neck

WHERE YOU SHOULD FEEL IT
Arms, lower back, upper back, neck, and abdominals

STARTING POSITION
Standing

Place your hands on your lower stomach with your elbows open to the sides. With the aid of your hands, lift the lower stomach in and up.

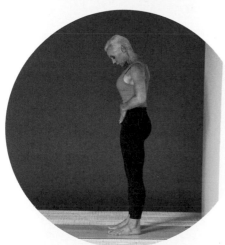

1 Inhale and reach your chin toward your chest, moving only your head and neck. Gaze at your hands.

2 Exhale and return to upright. Roll your shoulders back three times in a circle by lifting your shoulders toward your ears, together behind you, down to your sides, and forward to hollow the chest.

3 Inhale and reach your chin toward your chest, moving only your head and neck. Then continue to round forward, deepening the stretch to feel the ribs and spine stretch.

4 Exhale and return to upright. Repeat steps 2 and 3, rounding forward a little deeper. Repeat once more.

5 Let your arms lengthen down by your sides. Execute a Post-Shower Postural Check-In (page 93).

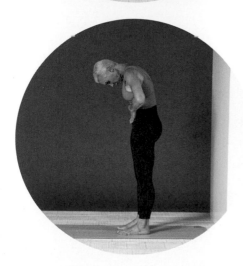

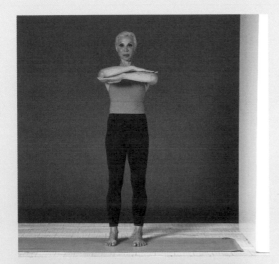

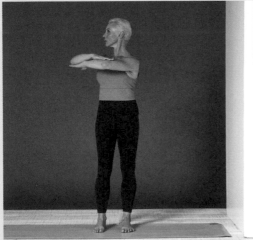

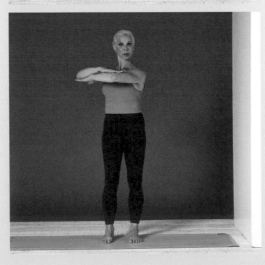

GENIE TWIST

TRY IT FOR
Lower back, upper back, shoulders, and neck

WHERE YOU SHOULD FEEL IT
Inner thighs, hips, waist, ribs, lower back, and neck

STARTING POSITION
Standing
Stand with your back close to the wall for safety. Position your legs sit-bone-width apart and parallel; your feet should face forward.

1 Bend your knees softly so that your knees are over your second toes. Lift your arms to chest height, arms in line with your shoulders and palms facing down.

2 Fold your arms at shoulder height, fingertips to elbows. Then, without moving the pelvis or hips, twist to the right.

3 Stay in the twist and turn your head to the left, chin toward the left shoulder, then twist and turn your head to the right, chin toward the right shoulder. Repeat the head turning left and right twice.

4 Untwist returning to face center. Repeat the twist to the left. Untwist back to center.

5 Switch which arm is on top, then repeat the twist in both directions.

6 Untwist and return to face center. Unfold your arms and extend them forward at chest height. Arms are in line with your shoulders and palms face down. Lower your arms to your sides. Execute a Post-Shower Postural Check-In (page 93).

➤➤ **TOO CHALLENGING?**
See opposite page for an easier option.

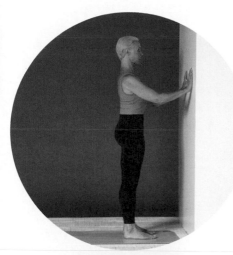

ALTERNATIVE STRETCH
TWIST WITH ONE HAND ON THE WALL

TRY IT FOR
Lower back, upper back, shoulders, and neck

WHERE YOU SHOULD FEEL IT
Inner thighs, hips, waist, ribs, lower back, shoulders, and neck

STARTING POSITION
Standing
Place your hands on the wall in front of you, fingertips at shoulder height and pointed up, palms flat. Bend your elbows and point them down. Zip up those tight jeans! Place your legs sit-bone-width apart and parallel, with toes facing forward and knees facing the wall.

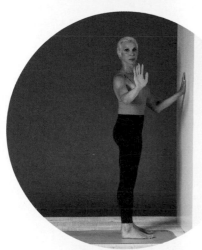

1 Without moving from the hips down, twist your shoulders to the right with a bent arm and palm facing out, your gaze following your hand. Hold the twist for three counts.

2 Return your hand to the wall and repeat on the other side.

3 Repeat, alternating sides three times. Lower your arms to your sides and execute a Post-Shower Postural Check-In (page 93).

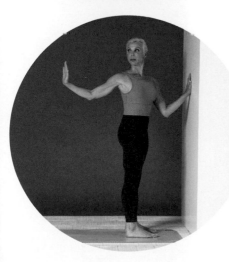

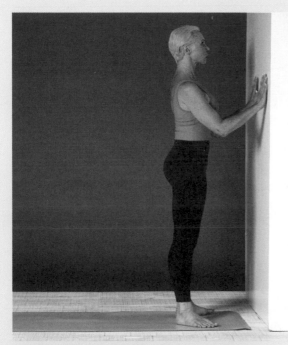

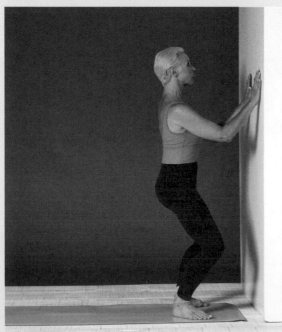

TURNED-OUT SQUATS

TRY IT FOR

Knees, ankles, lower back, and hips

WHERE YOU SHOULD FEEL IT

Thighs, glutes, calves, and hips

STARTING POSITION

Standing

Place your hands on the wall in front of you at shoulder height, palms flat and fingers pointed up. Bend your elbows and point them down. Zip up those tight jeans! Position your legs sit-bone-width apart and turned out slightly at a 45-degree angle, with feet facing the same direction, and point your knees over your toes.

1 Inhale with your stomach pulled in to protect your spine. Bend your knees so that they extend over, but not past, your toes. Try to keep your heels down, although they may lift. Hold squat for five counts.

2 Exhale and extend the legs. Repeat twice.

3 Inhale and straighten your knees, stomach pulled in to protect the spine, and arms lengthening down by your sides. Execute a Post-Shower Postural Check-In (page 93).

➥ TOO CHALLENGING?

See opposite page for an easier option.

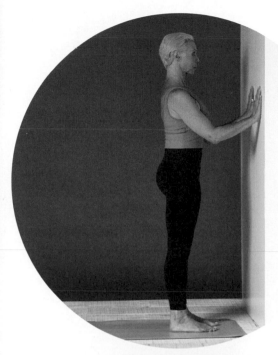

ALTERNATIVE STRETCH
PARALLEL SQUATS

TRY IT FOR
Knees, ankles, lower back, and hips

WHERE YOU SHOULD FEEL IT
Thighs, glutes, calves, and hips

STARTING POSITION
Standing
Place your hands on the wall in front of you at shoulder height, fingers pointed up and palms flat. Bend your elbows and point them down. Zip up those tight jeans! Position your legs so they are sit-bone-width apart and parallel, feet facing forward and knees facing the wall.

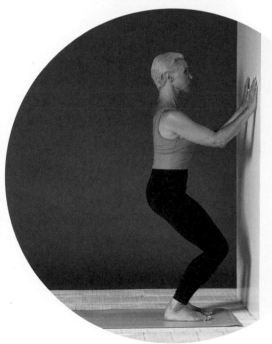

1 Inhale, pulling your stomach in to protect your spine. Bend your knees so they extend over, but not past, your toes. Try to keep your heels down, although they may lift. Hold squat for five counts.

2 Exhale and extend your legs. Repeat twice.

3 Inhale and straighten your knees, stomach pulled in to protect the spine, and arms lengthened down by your sides. Execute a Post-Shower Postural Check-In (page 93).

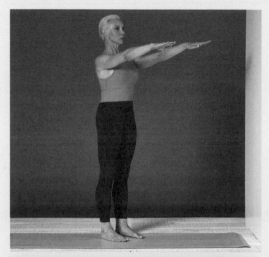

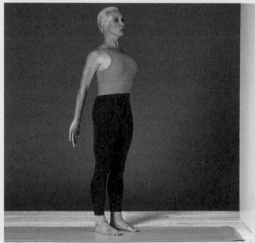

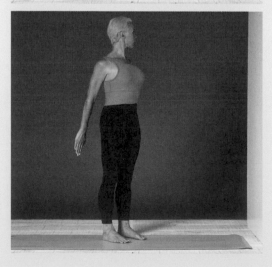

CHEST EXPANSION WITH HEAD TURN

TRY IT FOR
Neck, shoulder, and chest tightness

WHERE YOU SHOULD FEEL IT
Chest, shoulders, and neck

STARTING POSITION
Standing
Stand with your legs a little more than sit-bone-width apart. Heels should be under the hips, feet pointing forward. Arms are by your sides, with soft elbows.

1 Lift your arms in front of you to shoulder height, palms facing the floor.

2 Inhale and lower both arms simultaneously to pass your side body. Expand your chest and bring your shoulder blades together. Turn your head to the right. Hold for three counts, then exhale and face forward.

3 Inhale and turn your head to the left. Hold for three counts, then exhale and face forward.

4 Inhale and lift your arms to shoulder height, then repeat, beginning with a head turn to the left. Execute a Post-Shower Postural Check-In (page 93).

➤➤TOO CHALLENGING?
See opposite page for an easier option.

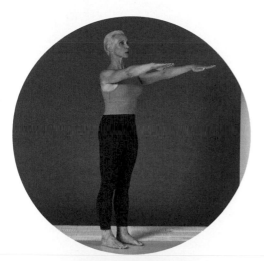

CHEST EXPANSION WITHOUT HEAD TURN

TRY IT FOR
Neck, shoulder, and chest tightness

WHERE YOU SHOULD FEEL IT
Chest, shoulders, and neck

STARTING POSITION
Standing
Stand with your legs a little more than sit-bone-width apart, with your heels under your hips and feet pointing forward. Let your arms hang by your sides, elbows soft.

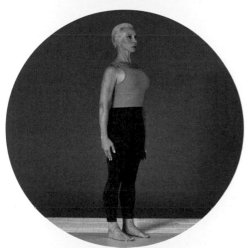

1 Lift your arms out in front of you to shoulder height, with palms facing the floor. Inhale and lower both arms simultaneously to pass the side of your body. Expand your chest and bring your shoulder blades together.

2 Exhale and lift your arms to shoulder height, palms facing the floor.

3 Repeat twice, then execute a Post-Shower Postural Check-In (page 93).

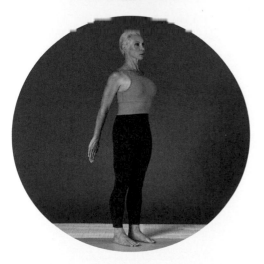

Seated Chair Stretches

You'll need two things for this set of stretches:

1. <u>A sturdy high-backed chair</u>. I prefer a kitchen chair made of wood. You may use a small seat cushion for comfort, as long as the cushion is secured to the chair and doesn't slide.

2. <u>A standard-size bath towel</u>, which can be sized from 20 x 40 inches to 28 x 54 inches. Don't use a bath sheet or plush towel. Holding a towel will build hand strength with any shoulder and wrist stretches.

Similar to the bed stretches, this series will gradually awaken your body to help you move with ease from seated to standing.

And, just like the Post-Shower Stretches, the Postural Check-In for this series is also the starting position (except where noted). Sit in the center of the chair seat unless directed otherwise. Work at the 70% level for maximum benefits and safety in this and all the movements. If you're shorter and your feet aren't flat on the floor, place yoga blocks underneath your feet. You can also do these seated moves in the bathroom, after your post-shower stretches—just have your chair ready!

SEATED POSTURAL CHECK-IN

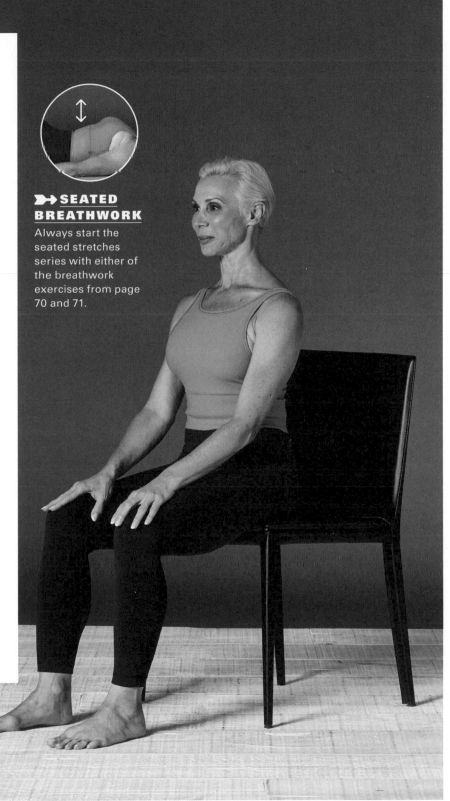

1 Sit upright with shoulders over your hips and legs a little more than sit-bone-width apart. Bend your knees at a 90-degree angle, with your knees over your heels. Point your feet forward with the arches of your feet lifted (keep your big toe on the floor and shift your feet so the outer edges are more in contact with the floor).

2 Let your arms hang by your sides, elbows soft. Then place your hands on your thighs and relax your arms.

3 Pull your stomach toward your spine as if zipping up a tight pair of jeans. Lift your navel toward your spine to protect your lower back.

4 Draw your shoulder blades toward each other behind you. Broaden your collarbones and soften your ribs as if a corset supports them.

5 Lengthen your neck as if a string is attached from the crown of your head to the ceiling, lifting you, and bring your gaze straight ahead.

6 Take a full deep breath, smile, and enjoy this feeling.

➤➤ SEATED BREATHWORK
Always start the seated stretches series with either of the breathwork exercises from page 70 and 71.

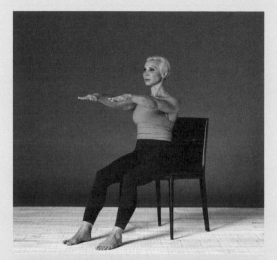

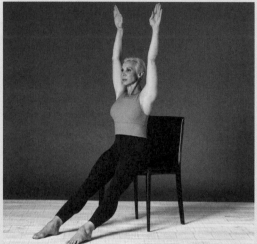

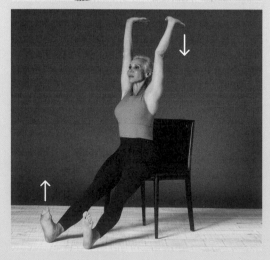

FULL-BODY STRETCH WITH ARM ARCS

TRY IT FOR
Stiffness through the entire body

WHERE YOU SHOULD FEEL IT
Entire body

STARTING POSITION
Seated

1 On a deep inhalation, lift your arms to shoulder height and then overhead. As the arms arc, extend your legs straight out from the chair. Spread your fingers and toes and flex your feet and hands.

2 Stretch in two directions, pushing through your heels and pressing your palms upward. Hold the stretch for three counts.

3 Exhale and stop flexing your hands and feet. Bend your knees to the Starting Position. Simultaneously, lift both arms to the ceiling.

4 Lower your arms to shoulder height, then lower your arms to your sides. Execute a Seated Postural Check-In (page 113).

➤➤ TOO CHALLENGING?
See opposite page for an easier option.

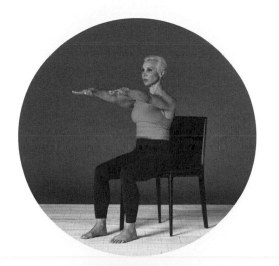

ALTERNATIVE STRETCH
TWO-WAY STRETCH

TRY IT FOR
Stiffness through the entire body

WHERE YOU SHOULD FEEL IT
Entire body

STARTING POSITION
Seated

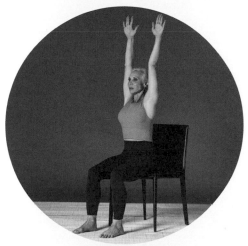

1 On a deep inhalation, lift your arms to shoulder height and then overhead toward the ceiling. Spread your fingers and toes.

2 Flex your feet and hands. Pull your toes toward your knees and press your palms away from you, toward the ceiling. Stretch in two directions, holding the stretch for three counts.

3 Exhale and stop flexing your hands and feet. Relax everything! Repeat three times, then execute a Seated Postural Check-In (page 113).

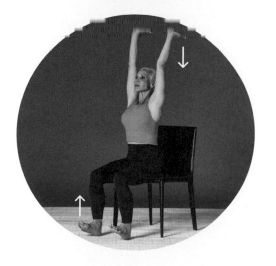

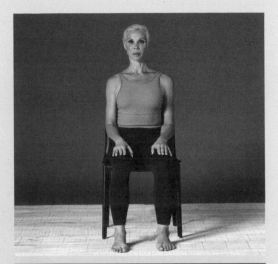

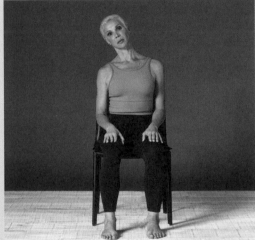

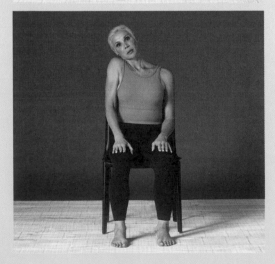

EAR AND SHOULDER TAPS

TRY IT FOR
Neck and shoulders

WHERE YOU SHOULD FEEL IT
Sides of neck

STARTING POSITION
Seated

1 Without straining, tip your right ear toward your right shoulder. Keep your head tilted, and raise and lift your right shoulder toward your ear three times.

2 Lift your head so it's upright, and relax your shoulders.

3 Tip your left ear toward your left shoulder. Keep your head tilted and raise and lift your left shoulder toward your ear three times.

4 Return your head upright and execute a Seated Postural Check-In (page 113).

➤➤ TOO CHALLENGING?
See opposite page for an easier option.

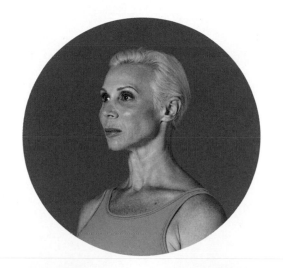

ALTERNATIVE STRETCH
YES AND NO

TRY IT FOR
Neck and shoulders

WHERE YOU SHOULD FEEL IT
Nook

STARTING POSITION
Seated

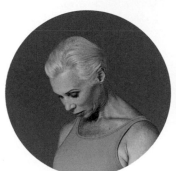
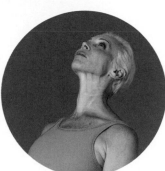

YES EXERCISE

1 Reach your chin toward your chest, but don't close your throat. Pause to gently stretch the neck for one count.

2 Return your head to center, gaze forward.

3 Lift your chin; you will be looking at the ceiling.

4 Return your head to center, keeping your gaze on the ceiling, and pause for one count. Resume the starting position.

5 Repeat the entire stretch two times. Execute a Seated Postural Check-In (page 113).

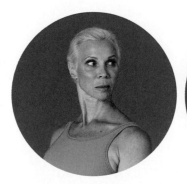
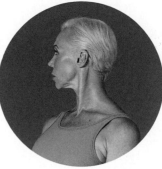

NO EXERCISE

1 Turn your head to the right as the left ear gently reaches forward. Hold for three counts. Return to center.

2 Turn your head to the left, as the right ear gently reaches forward. Hold for three counts.

3 Repeat to the right and left three times.

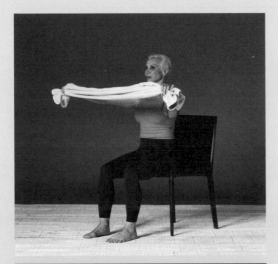

SEATED CHEERLEADER TOWEL STRETCH

TRY IT FOR
Shoulders and neck

WHERE YOU SHOULD FEEL IT
Shoulders, upper back, and arms

STARTING POSITION
Seated

Roll your bath towel lengthwise, the thinnest and longest way it can be rolled. Hold the towel with your hands as wide as possible, palms down, so it's taut across your lap.

1 On a deep inhalation, lift your arms to chest height and then overhead. Then exhale and bring your shoulder blades together. Inhale and bring your right arm to your ear. Lower your left arm to the side, keeping the towel taut.

2 Switch: Bring your left arm to your left ear and lower your right arm to the side. Exhale, then center the towel overhead.

3 Move your hands one inch closer together and repeat the moves. Then repeat again, hands inching closer. Put the towel down and execute a Seated Postural Check-In (page 113).

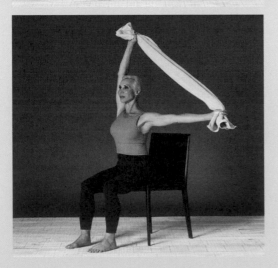

➤➤ TOO CHALLENGING?
See opposite page for an easier option.

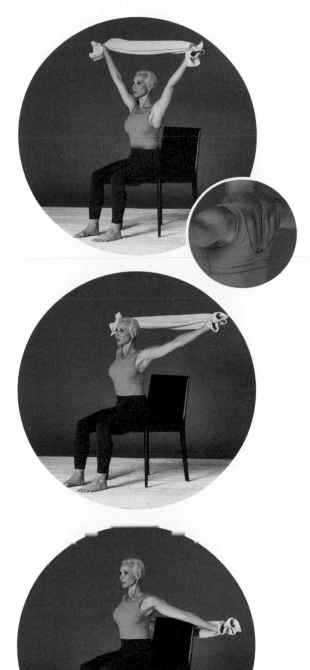

ALTERNATIVE STRETCH
TOWEL SHOULDER STRETCH

TRY IT FOR
Shoulders and neck

WHERE YOU SHOULD FEEL IT
Shoulders and upper back

STARTING POSITION
Seated

Roll your bath towel lengthwise, the thinnest and longest way it can be rolled. Hold the towel with your hands as wide as possible, palms down, so it's taut across your lap.

1 Inhale deeply. Lift your arms to chest height and then overhead. Exhale and bring your shoulder blades together and, if possible, reach your arms past and behind your head.

2 Inhale and stretch your arms gently up and back. Exhale and lower the towel to the starting position. Move your hands one inch closer and repeat the stretch. Continue to repeat, inching your hands closer together each time until your arms align with your shoulders. Put the towel down and execute a Seated Postural Check-In (page 113).

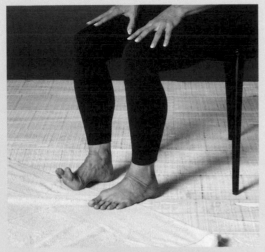

FOOT TOWEL STRETCH

TRY IT FOR
Ankles and feet

WHERE YOU SHOULD FEEL IT
Toes, foot arches, and ankles

STARTING POSITION
Seated

Spread the towel on the floor in front of you. Place your feet on the towel and your heels on the floor. Point your toes forward and make sure your knees are bent over your ankles, creating a 90-degree angle.

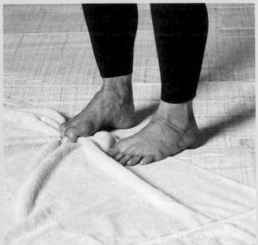

1 With your right foot, lift and spread your toes like a fan, and place the spread toes on the towel. Grasp the towel with your toes and pull your toes toward your heel. Your arch will lift off the towel. Relax your right foot.

2 Lift and fan the toes of your left foot and place them on the towel. Grasp the towel with your toes and pull your toes toward your heel; your arch will lift. Relax the left foot.

3 Repeat three times, alternating feet. Execute a Seated Postural Check-In (page 113).

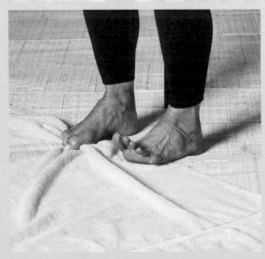

➡ TOO CHALLENGING?
See opposite page for an easier option.

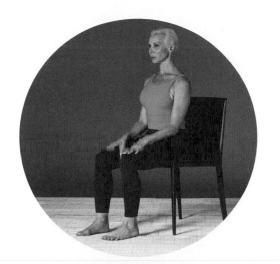

ALTERNATIVE STRETCH
FOUR PARTS OF THE FOOT

TRY IT FOR
Ankles and feet

WHERE YOU SHOULD FEEL IT
Thighs, ankles, and feet

STARTING POSITION
Seated

Sit with your legs a little more than sit-bone-width apart, feet flat on the ground. If you're tall enough, use the back of the chair to aid your back. If you're shorter and your feet aren't flat on the floor, place yoga blocks underneath your feet. Or sit in the center of the chair seat and place a pillow behind your back for support, if needed.

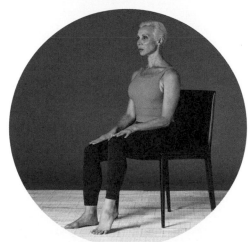

1 Without shifting your heel out or in, lift your right heel as if a high heel supports its center; let your knee rise straight up without swaying. Hold the lift for three counts. Don't lock your knee or arch your back.

2 Lift the knee higher and point your toes, so your foot hovers above the floor. Hold for three counts.

3 Slowly lower the ball of your foot to the floor with control. Hold the position for three counts, then slowly lower your heel to the floor with control.

4 Repeat with your left foot, then repeat three times, alternating feet, for a total of eight lifts. Execute a Seated Postural Check-In (page 113).

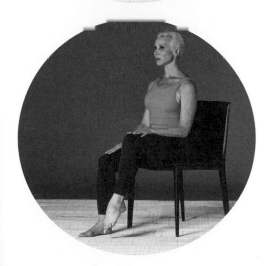

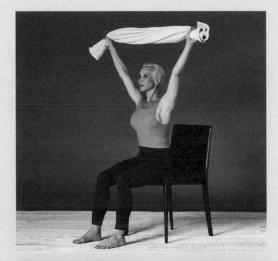

SEATED SIDE-TO-SIDE STRETCH WITH TOWEL

TRY IT FOR

Shoulders, waist, rib cage, lower back, and upper back

WHERE YOU SHOULD FEEL IT

Side body, waist, and shoulders

STARTING POSITION

Seated

Roll your bath towel lengthwise, the thinnest and longest way it can be rolled. Hold the towel with your hands as wide as possible, palms down, so it's taut across your lap.

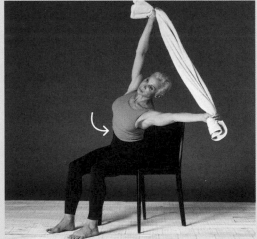

1 Inhale deeply and lift your arms to chest height, then overhead. Exhale and lift your arms as high as you can toward the ceiling to stretch your sides.

2 Inhale and stretch the right side of your body by reaching the towel to the left. Your head should remain centered between your arms. Support your back by pulling your stomach in.

3 Exhale and press the towel away from you while you bend your left elbow down and against your left side body to deepen the stretch. Inhale and extend the left arm out to the side.

4 Exhale and press the towel away from you to deepen the stretch.

5 On a deep inhalation, reverse the side bend to sit upright. Exhale and lift your arms as high as you can toward the ceiling to stretch your sides.

6 Inhale and stretch the left side of your body as above.

7 Repeat three times, alternating sides, and execute a Seated Postural Check-In (page 113).

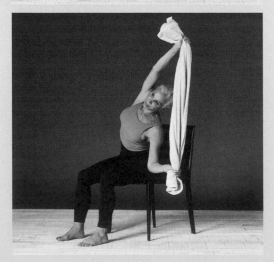

➔ TOO CHALLENGING?

See opposite page for an easier option.

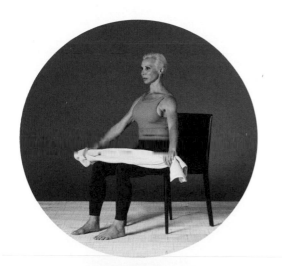

ALTERNATIVE STRETCH
SEATED SIMPLE SIDE-TO-SIDE STRETCH WITH TOWEL

TRY IT FOR
Shoulders, waist, rib cage, lower back, and upper back

WHERE YOU SHOULD FEEL IT
Side body, waist, and shoulders

STARTING POSITION
Seated

Sit in the center of your chair, legs a little more than sit-bone-width apart. Your toes should point forward, and your knees should be bent at 90 degrees and positioned over your ankles. Roll your bath towel lengthwise, the thinnest and longest way it can be rolled. Hold the towel with your hands as wide as possible, palms down, so it's taut across your lap.

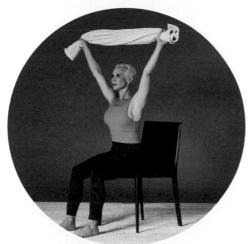

1 Inhale deeply and lift your arms to chest height, then overhead. Exhale and extend your arms as high as you can toward the ceiling to stretch your sides.

2 Inhale and stretch the right side of your body. Reach the towel over to the left, keeping your head centered between your arms. Support your back and keep your stomach pulled in.

3 Exhale and press the towel away from you to deepen the stretch. Then exhale deeply and reverse the side bend to sit upright.

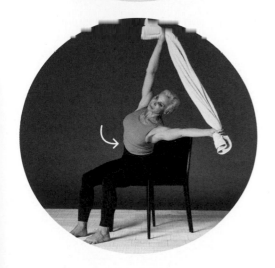

4 Exhale and lift your arms as high as you can toward the ceiling to stretch your sides. Then repeat steps 2 and 3 on the left, reversing the side bend on a deep inhalation to sit upright. Repeat three times, alternating sides. Execute a Seated Postural Check-In (page 113).

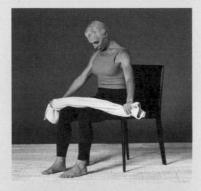

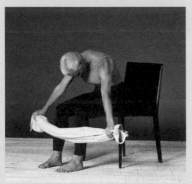

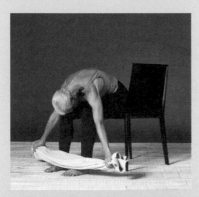

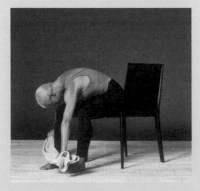

FORWARD STRETCH SEATED WITH TOWEL WITH TWIST

TRY IT FOR
Lower back, upper back, neck, and shoulders

WHERE YOU SHOULD FEEL IT
Arms, lower back, upper back, ribs, abdominals, and shoulders

STARTING POSITION
Seated

Roll your bath towel lengthwise, the thinnest and longest way it can be rolled. Hold the towel with your hands as wide as possible, palms down and arms straight, so it's taut across your lap.

1 Inhale deeply and lift your arms to chest height. Lower your head, bringing your gaze to the tops of your thighs. Exhale and roll your spine forward to place your hands on your knees, your head moving with your spine. The towel slides down your legs as you roll forward.

2 Slide the towel down your shins. Inhale and roll up your spine to bring your towel to your knees and your gaze to your thighs. Continue until you're sitting upright with your arms at chest height, gazing straight ahead.

3 Inhale deeply and twist your torso to the right, lowering your head to bring your gaze to the top of your right thigh. Exhale and roll your spine forward to place the towel on your right knee, moving your head with your spine. Slide the towel down your right shin.

4 Inhale and roll up your spine, bringing the towel to your right knee and your gaze to your right thigh. Continue rolling up until you're sitting upright, twisted over your right thigh, with your arms at chest height and your gaze straight ahead.

5 Turn your torso to face the center, then repeat the stretch to the left. Repeat the center-right-left sequence, and execute a Seated Postural Check-In (page 113).

➡️ TOO CHALLENGING?
See opposite page for an easier option.

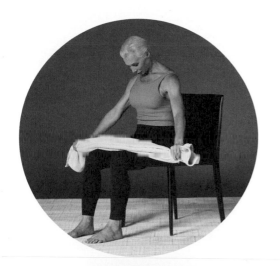

ALTERNATIVE STRETCH
FORWARD STRETCH SEATED WITH TOWEL

TRY IT FOR
Lower back, upper back, neck, and shoulders

WHERE YOU SHOULD FEEL IT
Arms, lower back, upper back, neck, abdominals, and shoulders

STARTING POSITION
Seated
Roll your bath towel lengthwise, the thinnest and longest way it can be rolled. Hold the towel with your hands as wide as possible, palms down and arms straight, so it's taut across your lap.

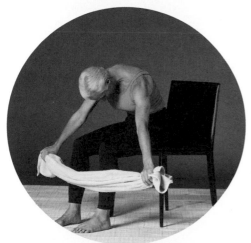

1 Inhale deeply and lift your arms to chest height. Lower your head to bring your gaze to the tops of your thighs. Exhale and slightly roll your spine forward to place the towel on your knees, head moving with the spine. The towel slides down your legs as you roll forward.

2 Slide the towel down your shins. Then inhale and roll your spine up, bringing your towel to your knees and your gaze to your thighs.

3 Continue rolling up until you're sitting upright with your arms at chest height and your gaze straight ahead. Repeat the stretch three times and execute a Seated Postural Check-In (page 113).

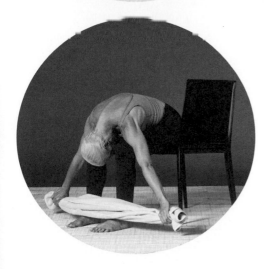

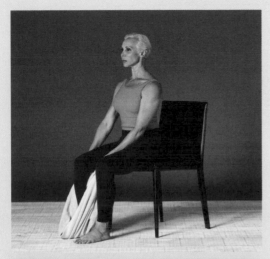

HAMSTRING STRETCH WITH TOWEL

TRY IT FOR
Lower back and hips

WHERE YOU SHOULD FEEL IT
Arms, lower back, back of the legs, hips, and ankles

STARTING POSITION
Seated

Fold the towel lengthwise, so it's about 6 inches wide. Place the towel under your right foot. Hold the ends of the towel with your hands at equal height and keep your back straight. The towel should be positioned under the ball and the arch of your foot.

1 Inhale, lift your right foot and bring your bent knee toward your chest. Exhale and straighten the leg. Inhale and hold this position for three counts.

2 Exhale and bend the leg. Inhale and lower the foot back to the start position.

3 Repeat three times with your right leg, then repeat the sequence three times with the left foot. Execute a Seated Postural Check-In (page 113).

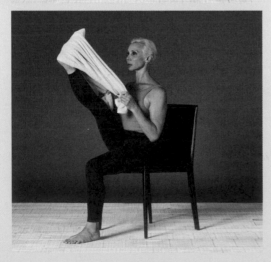

➤➤ TOO CHALLENGING?
See opposite page for an easier option.

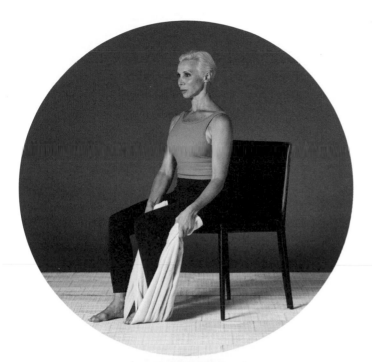

ALTERNATIVE STRETCH
SINGLE-KNEE LIFTS WITH TOWEL

TRY IT FOR
Lower back and hips

WHERE YOU SHOULD FEEL IT
Arms, lower back, hips, and ankles

STARTING POSITION
Seated

Fold the bath towel lengthwise, so it's about 6 inches wide. Place the towel under your right foot. Hold the ends of the towel with your hands at equal height and keep your back straight. The towel should be positioned under the ball and the arch of your foot.

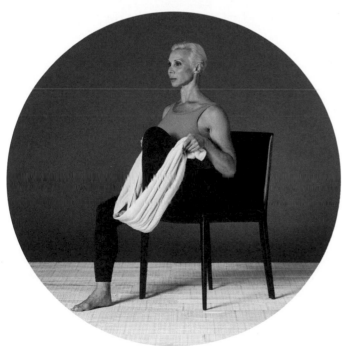

1 Inhale, lift your right foot with a bent knee, and bring your knee toward your chest. Exhale and hold this position for three counts.

2 Inhale and lower your foot back to the start position. Repeat three times with your right leg.

3 Repeat with your left foot, then execute a Seated Postural Check-In (page 113)

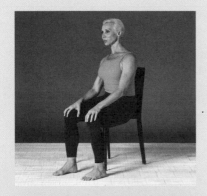

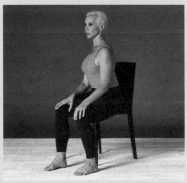

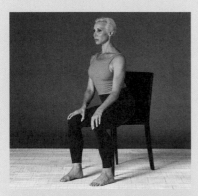

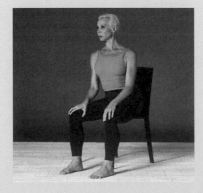

BOTTOMS UP, DOWN, AND AROUND

TRY IT FOR
Hips, waist, rib cage, and lower back

WHERE YOU SHOULD FEEL IT
Side body, waist, and hips

STARTING POSITION
Seated

Slide over in the chair so your right sit bone is off the side of the chair. Position your shoulders over your hips. If you feel unstable with one sit bone off the chair, hold on to a table or countertop for balance. Pull your stomach in to protect your back.

1 Shift the right hip straight back, then shift the right hip straight forward. Repeat three times.

2 Make a circle with the hip: Begin by shifting it straight back, then down, forward, and up. Repeat the circle, then reverse it, making two circles.

3 Repeat the stretch with the left side and execute a Seated Postural Check-In (page 113).

➡ TOO CHALLENGING?
See opposite page for an easier option.

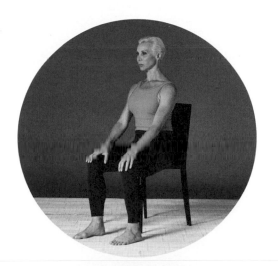

ALTERNATIVE STRETCH
BOTTOMS UP AND DOWN

TRY IT FOR

Hips, waist, rib cage, and lower back

WHERE YOU SHOULD FEEL IT

Side body, waistline, and hips

STARTING POSITION

Seated

Slide over in the chair so your right sit bone is off the side of the chair. Position your shoulders over your hips. If you feel unstable with one sit bone off the chair, hold on to a table or countertop for balance, and leave out the lifted arm variation. Pull your stomach in to protect your back.

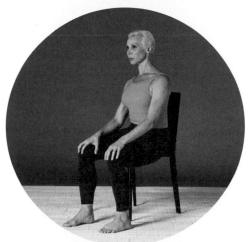

1 Lower the right hip to stretch the right side of your body, then lift the right hip, so both hip and sit bones are at the same height. Repeat. Then extend your right arm toward the ceiling while lowering the right hip, stretching your right side.

2 Lift the right hip, so both sit bones are at the same height. Repeat the lower and lift. Slide to the other side of the chair and repeat the stretch on the left side, then execute a Seated Postural Check-In (page 113).

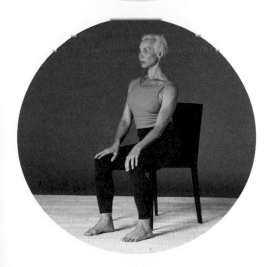

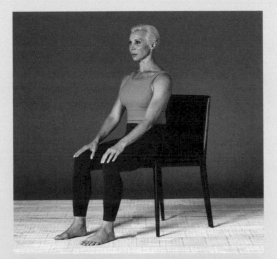

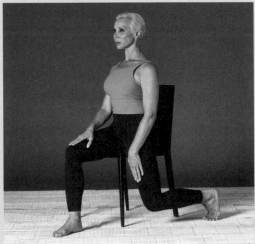

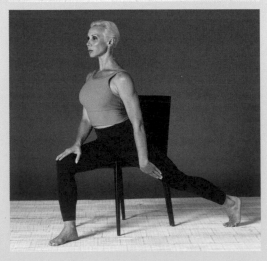

THIGH AND HIP STRETCH

TRY IT FOR

Hips

WHERE YOU SHOULD FEEL IT

Front of your hips and thighs

STARTING POSITION

Seated

Slide over in the chair so your right sit bone is off the side of the chair. Position your shoulders over your hips. If you feel unstable with one sit bone off the chair, hold on to a table or countertop for balance. Pull your stomach in to protect your back.

1 Pull your right foot straight back until your knee is under your hip; your heel will be lifted. Straighten your right leg and push your right heel back. Hold the stretch for three counts.

2 Bend your right knee and repeat the straightening and bending of the leg.

3 Return your right foot forward. Lift your right hip so both sit bones are at the same height.

4 Slide to the other side of the chair and repeat the stretch on the left side. Execute a Seated Postural Check-In (page 113).

➡➡ TOO CHALLENGING?

See opposite page for an easier option.

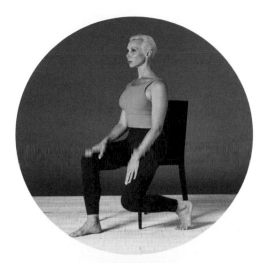

ALTERNATIVE STRETCH
THIGH AND HIP STRETCH WITH BENT LEGS

TRY IT FOR
Hips

WHERE YOU SHOULD FEEL IT
Front of your hips and thighs

STARTING POSITION
Seated
Slide over in the chair so your right sit bone is off the side of the chair. Position your shoulders over your hips. If you feel unstable with one sit bone off the chair, hold on to a table or countertop for balance. Pull your stomach in to protect your back.

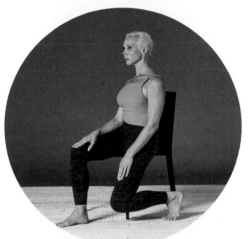

1 Move your right foot a few inches straight back, heel lifted.

2 Lower your right hip to stretch the right side of your body. Then lift your right hip, so both sit bones are at the same height. Repeat the lower and lift.

3 Move your right foot a few inches further back. Lower your right hip to stretch the right side of your body, then lift your right hip so that both sit bones are at the same height. Repeat the lower and lift before returning your right foot forward and lifting your right hip, so both sit bones are at the same height.

4 Slide to the other side of the chair and repeat the stretch on your left side. Execute a Seated Postural Check-In (page 113).

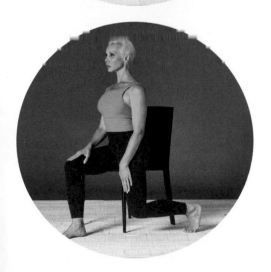

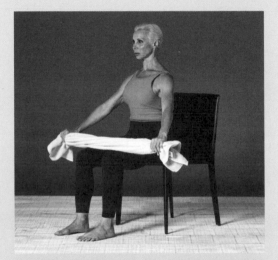

TOWEL TWIST

TRY IT FOR
Lower back, hips, and shoulders

WHERE YOU SHOULD FEEL IT
Legs, hips, front of the hips, waist, lower back, arms, and ribs

STARTING POSITION
Seated

Roll your bath towel lengthwise, the thinnest and longest way it can be rolled. Hold the towel taut across your thighs with your hands as wide as possible, palms down and arms straight.

1 Inhale deeply and lift your arms to chest height. Without moving your pelvis or hips, twist to the right, bringing the right upper arm back until you feel the stretch.

2 Stay in the twist and turn your head left and right three times.

3 Untwist and return to the face center. Repeat to the left. Repeat for a total of two twists in each direction. Execute a Seated Postural Check-In (page 113).

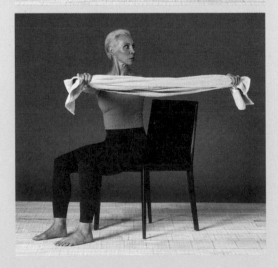

➡ **TOO CHALLENGING?**
See opposite page for an easier option.

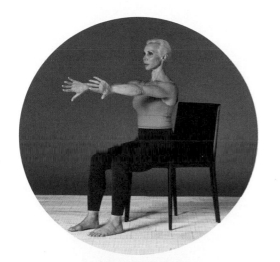

ALTERNATIVE STRETCH
HAND CLASP ARM AND SHOULDER STRETCH

TRY IT FOR
Lower back, hips, and shoulders

WHERE YOU SHOULD FEEL IT
Legs, hips, front of hips, waist, lower back, arms, ribs, wrists, and shoulders

STARTING POSITION
Seated

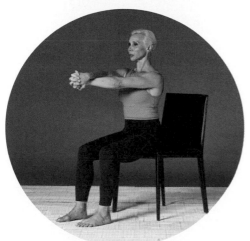

1 Inhale deeply and extend your arms forward at shoulder height. Spread your fingers and cross your wrists, right over left. Press palm to palm and interlace your fingers in the dominant grip (the natural way you interlace your fingers).

2 Keep your lower body still. Exhale as you twist your shoulders, ribs, and waist to the right. Squeeze the air out of your lungs, then inhale and return to center. Rotate until you feel the stretch. Repeat to the left.

3 Switch hands, so your other wrist is on top. Keep your lower body still and exhale as you twist your shoulders, ribs, and waist to the left. Squeeze the air out of your lungs, then inhale and return to center. Repeat.

4 Repeat the exercise, but this time with the non-dominant grip. Execute a Seated Postural Check-In (page 113).

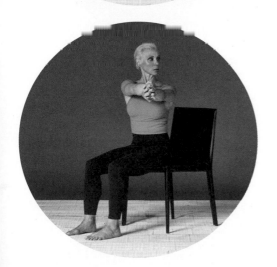

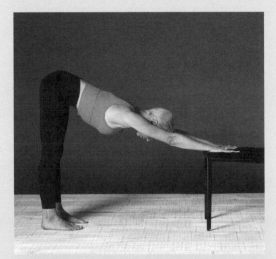

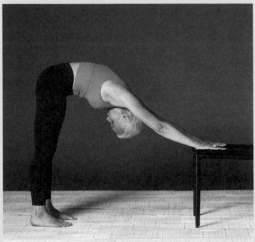

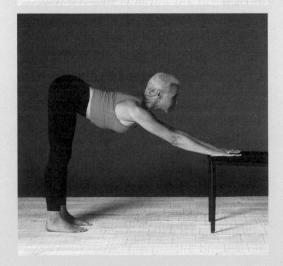

EXTENDED CAT

TRY IT FOR
Lower back, upper back, neck, shoulders, and hips

WHERE YOU SHOULD FEEL IT
Arms, lower back, upper back, shoulders, and abdominals

STARTING POSITION
Standing

By now you should feel ready to stand. Begin this stretch standing facing the chair, hands on the seat in front of you and in line with your shoulders. Keep your elbows soft and pointed toward your ribs, and your palms flat and fingers pointing forward. Zip up your imaginary tight jeans. Keep your legs sit-bone-width apart and parallel.

1 Walk your feet backward carefully, keeping a straight back as much as you can, without moving your hands. Your body should be in an inverted "L" position, shoulders in line with your wrists, arms straight, and your elbows soft. Point your fingers and toes forward, and keep your knees soft. Position your legs sit-bone-width apart.

2 Inhale and round your spine like a scared cat. Bring your gaze to your navel.

3 Exhale and, with your stomach pulled in to protect your spine, lift your chest and gently arch your back into the cow position.

4 Repeat the cat and cow three times. End in the cat position.

5 Draw your tailbone down toward the floor and let your hands slide off the chair as you roll up your spine to stand upright, shoulders over your hips. Execute a Standing Postural Check-In (page 137).

➡ TOO CHALLENGING?
See opposite page for an easier option.

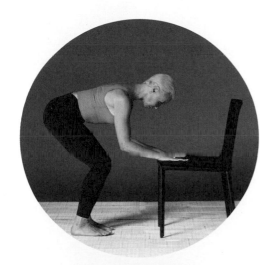

ALTERNATIVE STRETCH
CAT AND COW

TRY IT FOR
Lower back, upper back, neck, shoulders, and hips

WHERE YOU SHOULD FEEL IT
Arms, lower back, upper back, shoulders, and abdominals

STARTING POSITION
Standing

Stand facing the chair, hands on the seat in front of you and in line with your shoulders. Soften your elbows and point them toward your ribs. Keep your palms flat and fingers pointing forward. Zip up your imaginary tight jeans, and position your legs sit-bone-width apart and parallel.

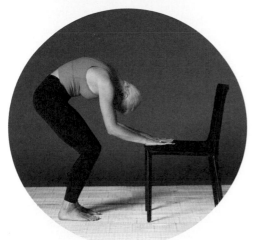

1 Inhale and round your spine. As you bring your gaze toward your navel, let your spine flex into a scared cat position. When your gaze reaches your navel, pause and press down with your hands. You should feel your back stretching.

2 Exhale, pull your stomach in to protect your spine, and lift your tailbone to reverse the action, lifting your chest and gently arching your back. Lift your chest and feel the stretch. Keep your navel lifted—don't allow your belly to hang.

3 Repeat three times. Stand upright. Execute a Standing Postural Check-In (page 137).

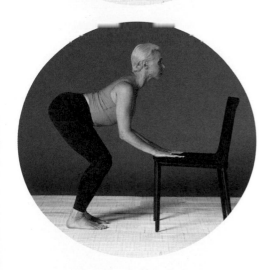

Standing Chair Stretches

Use a sturdy, high-backed chair for these exercises. If you don't have a high-backed chair, use a wall. When using the wall, place your fingertips at shoulder height. The leg positions will be the same. Except where noted, use the Postural Check-In at right at the beginning and end of each exercise.

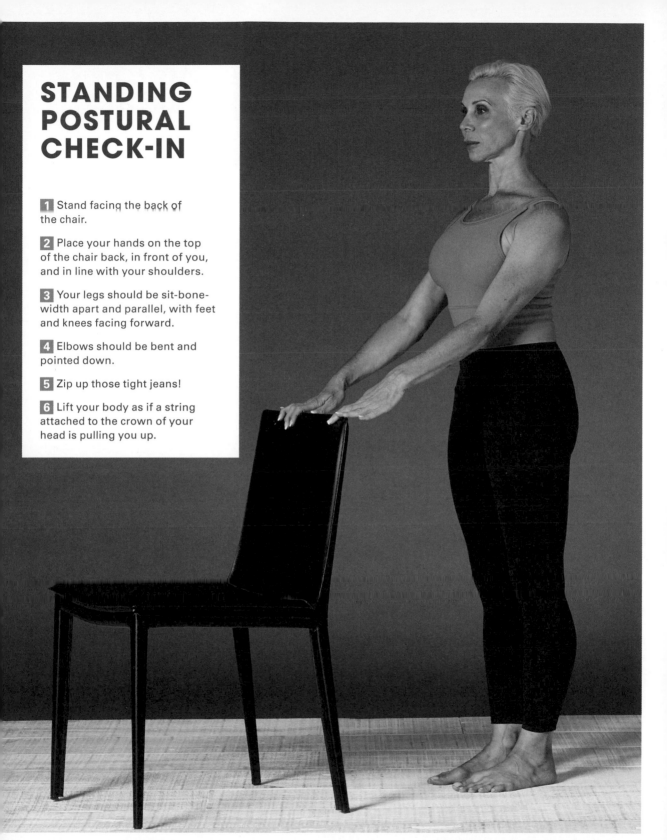

STANDING POSTURAL CHECK-IN

1 Stand facing the back of the chair.

2 Place your hands on the top of the chair back, in front of you, and in line with your shoulders.

3 Your legs should be sit-bone-width apart and parallel, with feet and knees facing forward.

4 Elbows should be bent and pointed down.

5 Zip up those tight jeans!

6 Lift your body as if a string attached to the crown of your head is pulling you up.

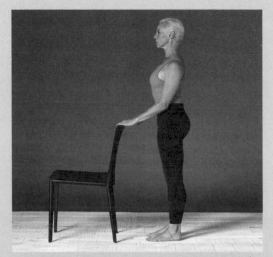

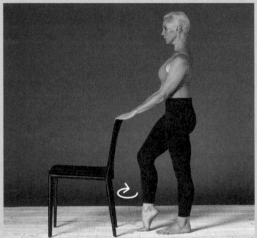

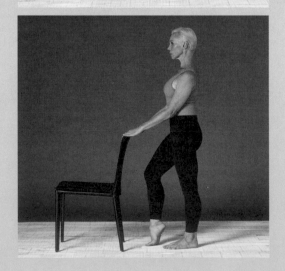

STANDING CHAIR ANKLE CIRCLES

TRY IT FOR
Ankles and feet

WHERE YOU SHOULD FEEL IT
Ankles and feet

STARTING POSITION
Standing behind chair

1 Bend your right knee and move your right foot forward and onto the ball of the foot, lifting your heel. Don't shift your hips or sink into one side; your shoulders and hips should form parallel lines.

2 Allowing your heel to lower and lift, circle the heel three times to the right and three times to the left.

3 Return to the start position and repeat with your left leg. Return to the start position and execute a Standing Postural Check-In (page 137).

➡ TOO CHALLENGING?
See opposite page for an easier option.

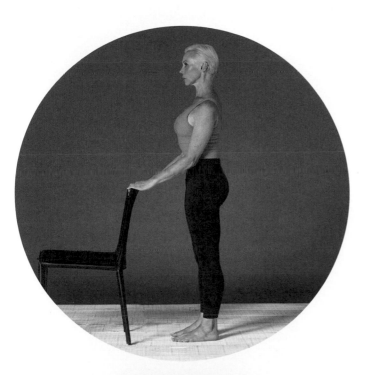

ALTERNATIVE STRETCH
HEEL LIFTS

TRY IT FOR
Ankles and feet

WHERE YOU SHOULD FEEL IT
Feet, ankles, thighs, and glutes

STARTING POSITION
Standing behind chair

1 Lift your heels straight up as if a hand is pushing them up, without shifting either heel out or in. Hold the lift for three counts. Don't lock your knees or arch your back, and spread your weight evenly across the balls of your feet.

2 With control, slowly lower your heels. Repeat the lift and lower three times, then execute a Standing Postural Check-In (page 137).

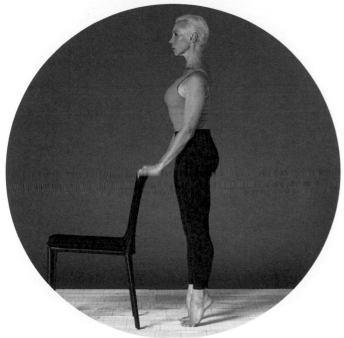

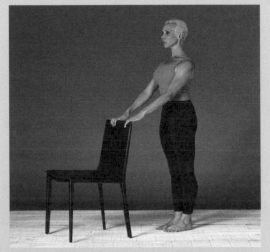

RUNNING IN PLACE, HEELS DOWN

TRY IT FOR
Ankles, feet, and knees

WHERE YOU SHOULD FEEL IT
Feet, ankles, thighs, and glutes

STARTING POSITION
Standing behind chair

1 Lift both heels. With the balls of your feet and toes still on the floor, bend your right knee—keeping the right heel lifted—while lowering the left heel with a straight leg.

2 Lift both heels. Then reverse, bending the left knee with the left heel lifted and lowering the right heel with a straight leg.

3 Repeat at a brisk pace for 10 to 20 "steps." Return to the start position and execute a Standing Postural Check-In (page 137).

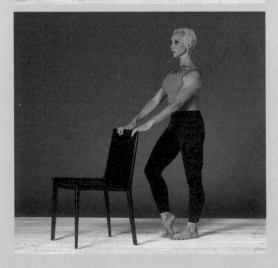

➡➡TOO CHALLENGING?
See opposite page for an easier option.

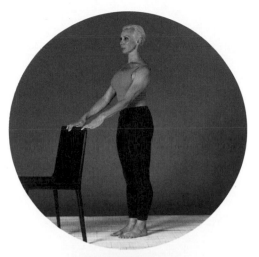

ALTERNATIVE STRETCH
FOUR PARTS OF THE FOOT

TRY IT FOR
Ankles, feet, and knees

WHERE YOU SHOULD FEEL IT
Feet, ankles, thighs, and glutes

STARTING POSITION
Standing behind chair

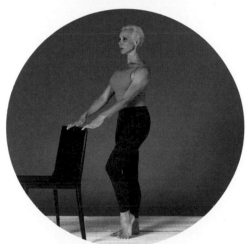

1 Point your right knee straight up and lift your right heel as if a high heel is supporting its center. Don't shift your heel out or in. Hold lift for three counts. Don't lock your knees or arch your back.

2 Lift your knee higher and point your toes. The toes should hover over the floor. Hold lift for three counts.

3 Slowly lower the ball of your right foot to the floor with control. Hold position for three counts.

4 Slowly lower your right heel to the floor with control. Repeat with the other foot, then repeat three more times, alternating feet. Return to the start position and execute a Standing Postural Check-In (page 137).

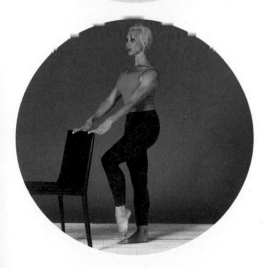

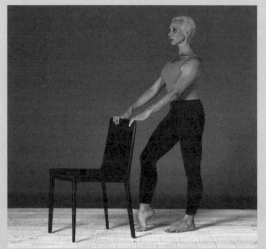

SINGLE-LEG SQUATS

TRY IT FOR

Knees, ankles, lower back, hips, and feet

WHERE YOU SHOULD FEEL IT

Thighs, glutes, calves, hips, and toes

STARTING POSITION

Standing behind chair

1 Bend your right knee and move that foot forward, lifting your heel so the ball of the foot is on the floor. Put about 70% of your body weight on the back or base leg. Don't shift your hips or lean to one side. Your shoulders and hips should form parallel lines.

2 Inhale and bend your knees, pulling your stomach in to protect your spine. Extend your knees over, but not past, your toes. Try to keep your back heel down, although it may lift.

3 Exhale and extend the base leg. The front leg will bend a little more but remain bent throughout. Repeat three times. Return to the start position and execute a Standing Postural Check-In (page 137).

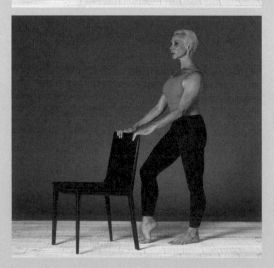

➡ TOO CHALLENGING?

See opposite page for an easier option.

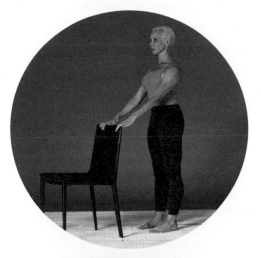

ALTERNATIVE STRETCH
SQUATS

TRY IT FOR
Knees, ankles, lower back, and hips

WHERE YOU SHOULD FEEL IT
Thighs, glutes, and calves

STARTING POSITION
Standing behind chair

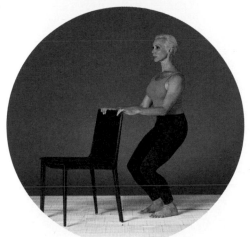

1 Point your fingers and toes forward, bend your knees, and position your legs sit-bone-width apart. Inhale and bend your knees, pulling in your stomach to protect your spine. Extend your knees over, but not past your toes. Try to keep your heels down, although they may lift.

2 Exhale and extend your legs so they are straight. Repeat three times.

3 Return to the start position. Execute a Standing Postural Check-In (page 137).

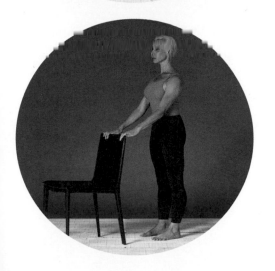

Wall Stretches

Use the wall for increased support and tactile feedback. Be sure the wall is free from obstruction and provides enough clear space for you to fully extend your arms.

STANDING AT THE WALL POSTURAL CHECK-IN

1 Stand upright a few inches away from the wall.

2 Your legs should be sit-bone-width apart and parallel, with feet and knees facing forward. Feel your feet on the ground.

3 Relax your arms by your sides.

4 Zip up those tight jeans!

5 Lift your body as if a string attached to the crown of your head is pulling you up.

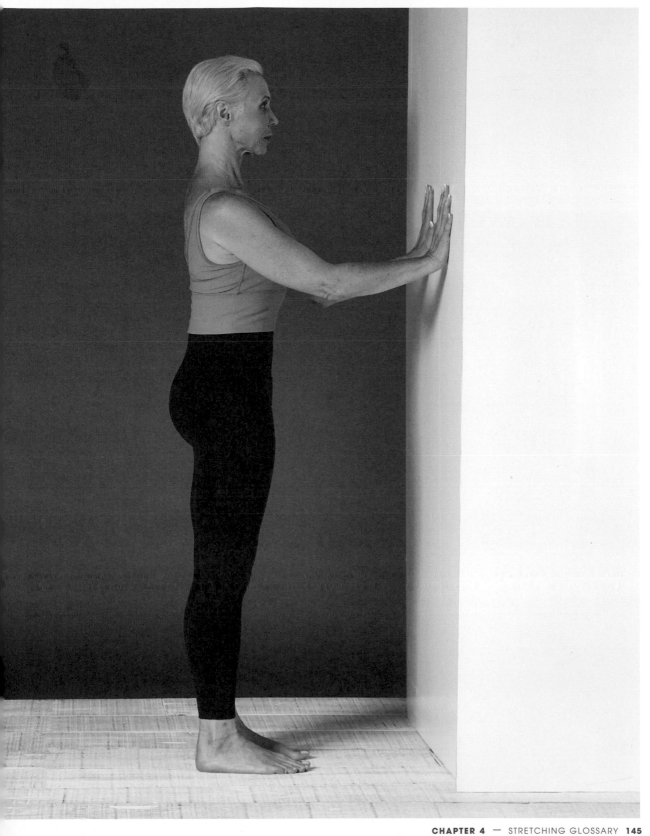

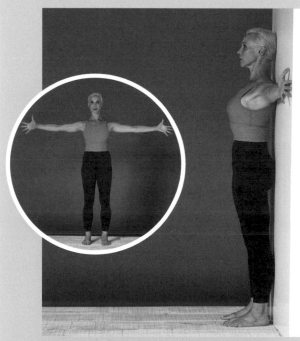

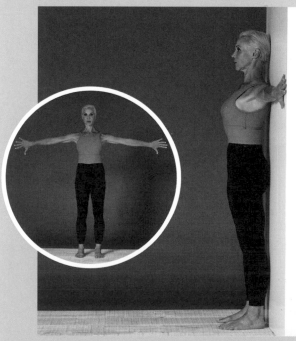

SPREAD EAGLE

TRY IT FOR
Shoulders, waist, rib cage, and upper back

WHERE YOU SHOULD FEEL IT
Chest, arms, and shoulders

STARTING POSITION
Standing

Stand with your back against an empty wall, arms at your sides. Your heels, glutes, upper back, and, if possible, the back of your head should touch the wall. Zip up your imaginary tight jeans to pull your stomach in and protect your spine.

1 Lift your arms so they are fully extended at shoulder height. Press your arms against the wall with hands flat, fingers long and spread, and your face forward. Press firmly for three counts. Feel your shoulder blades reaching together behind you, opening your chest.

2 Flip your hands so your palms are flat against the wall, fingers extended and spread out. Press firmly for three counts. Feel your shoulder blades reaching together behind you to open your chest.

3 Repeat the sets three times, then lower your arms to your sides. Execute a Standing at the Wall Postural Check-In (page 145).

➡ **TOO CHALLENGING?**
See opposite page for an easier option.

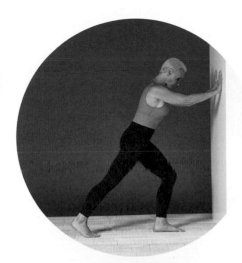

ALTERNATIVE STRETCH
PASSIVE SHOULDER STRETCHES

TRY IT FOR

Shoulders, waist, rib cage, lower back, upper back, and fingers

WHERE YOU SHOULD FEEL IT

Upper back, rib cage, waist, side body, hands, and shoulders

STARTING POSITION

Standing

Place your hands on the wall in front of you at shoulder height, palms flat and fingers pointing up, with your elbows touching your sides, soft and pointing down. Pull in your stomach to protect your back, and keep your back straight.

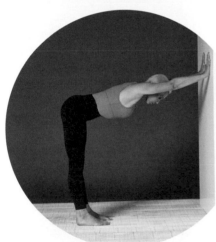

1 Walk your feet back carefully as far as possible, leaving your hands in place. Make an inverted "L" position with your arms, but don't pass your ears. Hold for three counts.

2 Walk back to the starting position and repeat three times.

3 Walk your feet back toward the wall to return to the start position, lower your arms to your sides and execute a Standing at the Wall Postural Check-In (page 146).

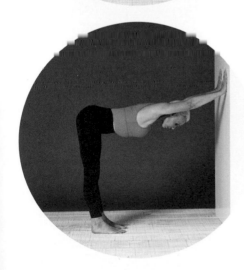

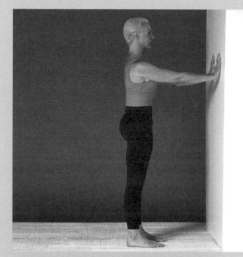

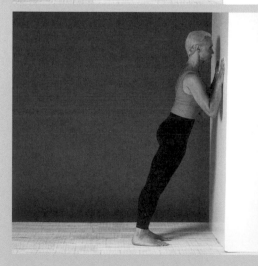

WALL PUSHUPS WITH ELBOWS BY RIBS

TRY IT FOR
Building and stretching the chest, shoulders, and arms

WHERE YOU SHOULD FEEL IT
Chest, shoulders, and arms

STARTING POSITION
Standing
Face the wall, legs as close together as possible. Place your hands on the wall in front of you at shoulder height, palms flat and fingers pointing up, with your elbows touching your sides, soft and pointing down. Pull in your stomach to protect your back, and keep your back straight.

1 Take two small steps away from the wall, ending with your legs together and parallel. Lift your heels. Bend your elbows, allowing them to brush your ribs. Keep your body still, like a plank. Hold this bent position for three counts.

2 Pull your stomach in to protect your spine and press into your hands to straighten your arms.

3 Repeat three times. Walk your feet toward the wall to return to the start position and lower your arms to your sides. Execute a Standing at the Wall Postural Check-In (page 145).

➡ TOO CHALLENGING?
See opposite page for an easier option.

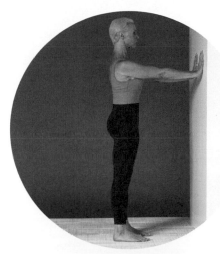

ALTERNATIVE STRETCH
WALL PUSHUPS WITH ELBOWS OUT

TRY IT FOR
Chest, shoulders, and arms

WHERE YOU SHOULD FEEL IT
Chest, shoulders, and arms

STARTING POSITION
Standing

Face the wall, legs as close together as possible. Place your hands on the wall in front of you at shoulder height, palms flat and fingers pointing up, with your elbows touching your sides, soft and pointing down. Pull in your stomach to protect your back, and keep your back straight.

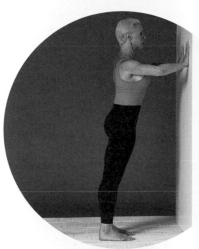

1 Take two small steps back, away from the wall, ending with legs together and parallel to each other. Bend your elbows out to the side. Keep your body still, as if you're performing a plank. Hold the bent-elbow position for three counts.

2 Pull your stomach in to protect your spine, and press into your hands to straighten your arms.

3 Repeat three times, then walk your feet toward the wall to return to the start position, lowering your arms to your sides. Execute a Standing at the Wall Postural Check-In (page 145).

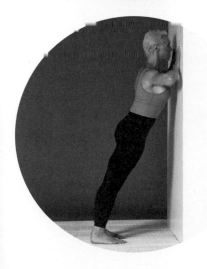

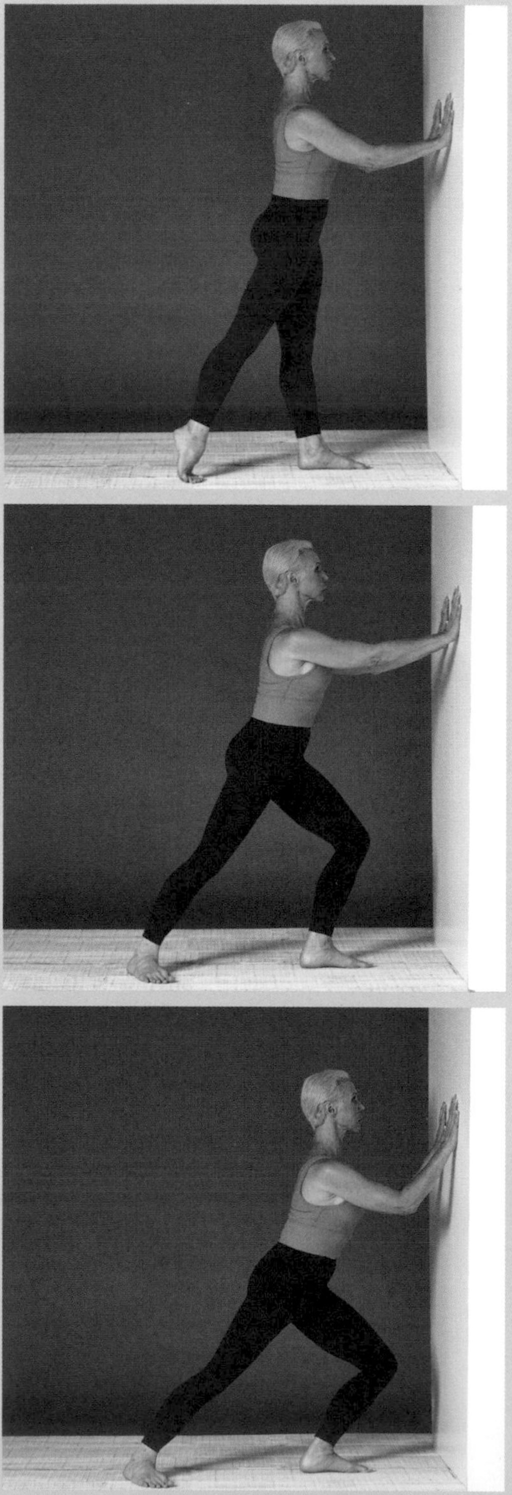

ONE-LEG BACK LUNGE

TRY IT FOR

Knee, ankles, hips, and feet

WHERE YOU SHOULD FEEL IT

Thighs, glutes, calves, hips, and toes

STARTING POSITION

Standing

Stand facing the wall, about 1 foot away from it, legs sit-bone-width apart and parallel. Your heels should be under your sit bones, and your toes should point forward; keep your knees straight but not locked. Arms are by your sides, with soft elbows. Your gaze is forward.

1 Lift your arms in front of you to shoulder height and place your hands on the wall. Keep both legs in line with your hips and step your right leg back, keeping the heel lifted. The heel should be in line with its hip or sit bone and the center of the ball of the foot.

2 Turn the back leg out slightly and lower your heel. Bend your front leg as you lower your heel, putting your foot at a 45-degree angle. Keep your shoulders and hips as parallel as possible to the wall.

3 Maintaining a lifted torso, with shoulders over hips, deepen your front leg's bend. Move your torso closer to the wall. Press the outer edge of the back foot and its large toe down. Hold the stretch.

4 Release the tension, then repeat the stretch three times.

5 Switch your legs and repeat the series on the second side. Then step your back leg forward to stand with your legs a little more than sit-bone-width apart. Lower your arms to your sides to finish and execute a Standing at the Wall Postural Check-In (page 145).

TOO CHALLENGING?

See opposite page for an easier option.

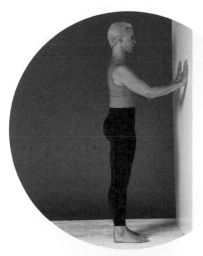

ALTERNATIVE STRETCH
ONE-LEG BACK SQUAT

TRY IT FOR
Knees, ankles, hips, and feet

WHERE YOU SHOULD FEEL IT
Knees, ankles, hips, and feet

STARTING POSITION
Standing
Stand facing the wall, 1 foot away from it. Place your legs sit-bone-width apart and parallel, heels under sit bones, toes pointing forward, and knees straight but not locked. Let your arms hang by your sides, with soft elbows. Direct your gaze forward.

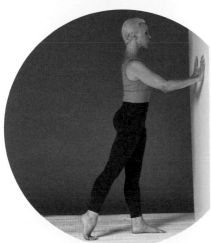

1 Raise your arms to shoulder height in front of you and place your hands on the wall. Keep both legs in line with your hips, and move your right leg back, lifting your heel. Keep your heel in line with its sit bone and with the center of the ball of your foot. Shift your body weight to the front leg, with shoulders and hips parallel.

2 With your stomach pulled in to protect your spine, bend your front knee so it extends over but not past your toes, and bend your back knee directly down toward the floor. Keep your knees facing front. Exhale and straighten your legs.

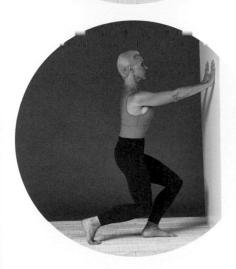

3 Repeat three times, then step the back leg forward and repeat on the second side. Step your back leg forward to stand with your legs a little more than sit-bone-width apart. Lower your arms to your sides to finish, and execute a Standing at the Wall Postural Check-In (page 145).

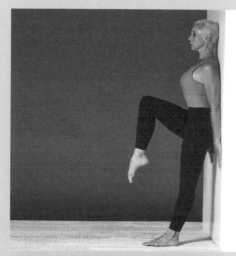

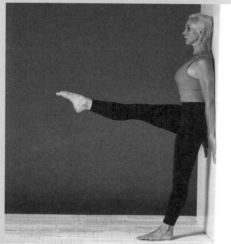

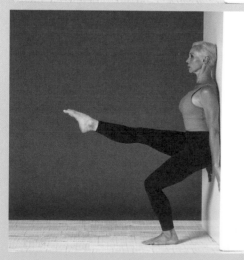

SINGLE-LEG SQUATS

TRY IT FOR
Knees, ankles, lower back, and hips

WHERE YOU SHOULD FEEL IT
Thighs, glutes, calves, and abdominals

STARTING POSITION
Standing

Stand with your back to the wall, keeping your legs sit-bone-width apart and parallel and knees facing forward. Press the back of your torso against the wall. Walk your feet 6 to 8 inches out in front of you, and soften your knees so that your back is flush with the wall. Your hips, knees, second toes, and the centers of your heels should be in alignment with each other.

1 Bend your right knee and lift your foot without shifting your hips or sinking into one side. Your shoulders and hips should form parallel lines. Straighten your right leg.

2 With your stomach pulled in to protect your spine, inhale and bend your bottom knee so that your legs form a 90-degree angle. The knee should not extend past the toes. Try to keep your back heel down, although it may lift.

3 Exhale and extend the base leg to the start position and place the right foot down.

4 Lift your left foot and repeat the squat with your left foot lifted.

5 Repeat, alternating legs, three times. Straighten your legs and walk your feet back to the wall to stand upright. Step away from the wall and execute a Standing at the Wall Postural Check-In (page 145).

➡➡ TOO CHALLENGING?
See opposite page for an easier option.

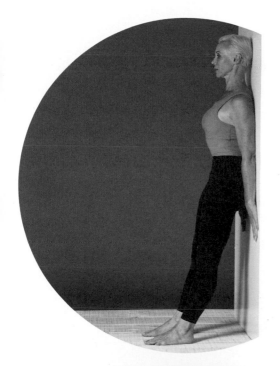

ALTERNATIVE STRETCH
WALL SQUATS

TRY IT FOR
Knees, ankles, hips, feet, and lower back

WHERE YOU SHOULD FEEL IT
Thighs, glutes, calves, and abdominals

STARTING POSITION
Standing

Stand with your back to the wall, keeping your legs sit-bone-width apart and parallel and knees facing forward. Press the back of your torso against the wall. Walk your feet 6 to 8 inches out in front of you, and soften your knees so that your back is flush with the wall. Your hips, knees, second toes, and the centers of your heels should be in alignment with each other.

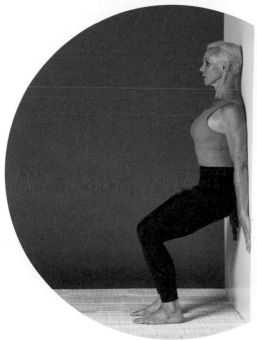

1 Inhale and bend your knees so that your legs form a 90-degree angle. Pull your stomach in to protect your spine. Your knees should not pass your toes. Try to keep your heels down, although they may lift. Slide your torso down the wall and hold for four counts.

2 Exhale and extend the legs, sliding your torso up the wall. Repeat three times.

3 Straighten your legs and walk your feet back to the wall to stand upright. Step away from the wall and execute a Standing at the Wall Postural Check-In (page 145).

© 2023 by Hearst Magazines, Inc.

Book design by Karina Ponce and Gillian MacLeod

Library of Congress Cataloging-in-Publication Data is on file with the publisher.

ISBN 978-1-955710-20-6

Printed in China

4 6 8 10 9 7 5 hardcover

HEARST

Photo Credits

COVER PHOTOGRAPHY
PHILIP FRIEDMAN

INTERIOR PHOTOGRAPHY
ADOBE STOCK: 12, 17, 18, 22, 26, 27, 35, 36, 42;

PHILIP FRIEDMAN: 9, 10, 21, 24, 28-34, 40, 43-153, 159;

GETTY IMAGES/ COMPASSIONATE EYE FOUNDATION/STONE: 14

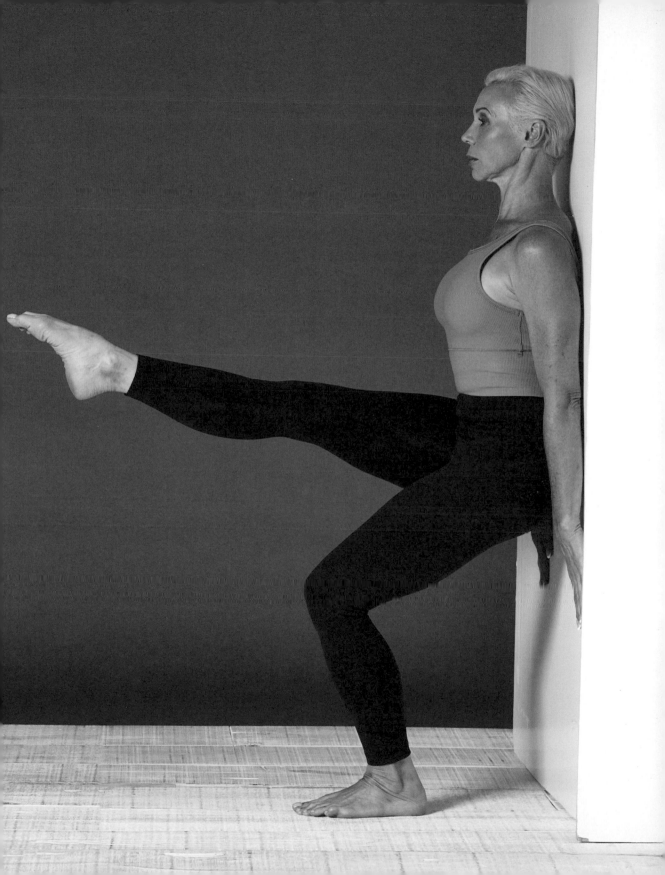

Thank you!

For purchasing Stretch Away Pain

Visit our online store to find more great products
from Prevention and save 20% off your next purchase.

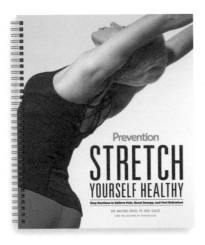
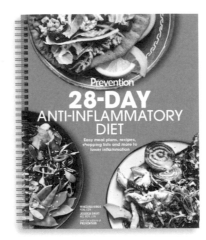
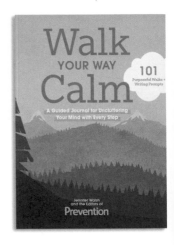

Your feedback is important to us! Scan the QR
to leave a review for **Stretch Away Pain**.

shop.prevention.com

*Exclusions Apply

H E A R S T